A Clinician's Brief Guide to the Mental Health Act

Fifth edition

A Clinician's Brief Guide to the Mental Health Act

Tony Zigmond
Consultant General Adult Psychiatrist, RCPsych Lead on Mental Health Law

Nick Brindle
Consultant Old Age Psychiatrist, Leeds and York Partnership NHS Foundation Trust

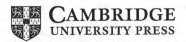

CAMBRIDGE
UNIVERSITY PRESS

University Printing House, Cambridge CB2 8BS, United Kingdom

One Liberty Plaza, 20th Floor, New York, NY 10006, USA

477 Williamstown Road, Port Melbourne, VIC 3207, Australia

314–321, 3rd Floor, Plot 3, Splendor Forum, Jasola District Centre, New Delhi – 110025, India

103 Penang Road, #05-06/07, Visioncrest Commercial, Singapore 238467

Cambridge University Press is part of the University of Cambridge.

It furthers the University's mission by disseminating knowledge in the pursuit of
education, learning, and research at the highest international levels of excellence.

www.cambridge.org
Information on this title: www.cambridge.org/9781009178303
DOI: 10.1017/9781009178297

First edition © The Royal College of Psychiatrists 2011
Second edition © The Royal College of Psychiatrists 2012
Third edition © The Royal College of Psychiatrists 2014
Fourth edition © The Royal College of Psychiatrists 2016
Fifth edition © The Royal College of Psychiatrists 2022

First published 2011, second, third and fourth editions published by Gaskell, The Royal College of
Psychiatrists. This fifth edition published by Cambridge University Press 2022

A catalogue record for this publication is available from the British Library.

Library of Congress Cataloging-in-Publication Data
Names: Zigmond, Tony, author. | Brindle, Nick, author.
Title: A clinician's brief guide to the Mental Health Act / Nick Brindle, Consultant Old Age Psychiatrist,
   Leeds and York Partnership NHS Foundation Trust; Tony Zigmond, Consultant General Adult
   Psychiatrist, RCPsych Lead on Mental Health Law.
Description: Fifth edition. | Cambridge, United Kingdom ; New York, NY : Cambridge University
   Press, 2022. | Includes bibliographical references and index.
Identifiers: LCCN 2022970036 (print) | LCCN 2022970037 (ebook) | ISBN 9781009178303 (paperback) |
   ISBN 9781009178297 (epub)
Subjects: LCSH: Mental health laws–England. | Mental health laws–Wales. | Great Britain. Mental
   Health Act 2007. | Great Britain. Mental Health Act 1983. | Mental health personnel–Great Britain–
   Handbooks, manuals, etc.
Classification: LCC KD3412 .Z54 2022 (print) | LCC KD3412 (ebook) | DDC 344.4104/4–dc23/eng/
   20220228
LC record available at https://lccn.loc.gov/2022970036
LC ebook record available at https://lccn.loc.gov/2022970037

ISBN 978-1-009-17830-3 Paperback

Contents

Preface to the First Edition

This is a 'how to' book. It is designed as an easy-to-read and interesting guide to understanding those parts of the Mental Health Act 1983 that clinicians need in their daily practice. It covers civil and court detentions, Community Treatment Orders, consent to treatment and giving written and oral evidence for Mental Health Tribunals. It also includes relevant aspects of the Human Rights Act 1998, the Mental Capacity Act 2005 (including the Deprivation of Liberty Safeguards) and illustrative case law. Although it should be of particular interest to doctors seeking approval under section 12 and doctors and other clinicians wishing to become Approved Clinicians in England, it will aid understanding of the processes for all users of the Mental Health Act.

More detailed guidance can be found in the Mental Health Act Codes of Practice, the *Reference Guide to the Mental Health Act* and many other texts.

Acts of Parliament and secondary legislation such as Statutory Instruments can be read and downloaded from the internet – but make sure that you are reading the updated (post-2007 amendments) version. These are readily searchable electronically, so to avoid cluttering the text with numbers we have not cited chapter and verse when using short quotations from Acts.

Acronyms and abbreviations abound in mental health legislation. We have used very few of these, but readers may find those listed on p. x useful when reading other sources.

Preface to the Second Edition

The Health and Social Care Act 2012 has made a number of amendments to the Mental Health Act 1983.

The most significant change, in relation to matters dealt with in this book, relates to the authorisation for prescribing medication for the treatment of mental disorder to patients on a Community Treatment Order. Other changes include amendments required by the abolition of Primary Care Trusts and Strategic Health Authorities and the establishment of the National Health Service (NHS) Commissioning Board and Clinical Commissioning Groups. The main issues are:

- the provision of section 117 aftercare;
- the duty to provide information to local social services about bed provision both for the admission to hospital of emergencies and for children and young people;
- the duty to provide information to the courts about bed availability;
- approval mechanisms for section 12 doctors and Approved Clinicians.

Other changes relate to the provision of Independent Mental Health Advocates and regulation of Social Workers.

Further amendments remove some of the powers of the Secretary of State. These include the authority to move detained patients from one high-secure hospital to another and to discharge detained NHS patients from private hospitals (the Act also removes the right of NHS bodies to do the latter). The power to grant 'pocket money' to in-patients is also removed in England (but not in Wales).

Preface to the Third Edition

The main statutory changes since the second edition are as follows.

- Primary legislation:
  - Mental Health (Discrimination) Act 2013. This reduces discrimination in three areas. It repeals section 141, which said that if a Member of Parliament (MP) was detained under the Mental Health Act for more than 6 months they would lose their seat (an MP has to be imprisoned for over a year to lose their seat, and doesn't lose their seat at all if unable to attend Parliament owing to physical illness). It amends the Juries Act 1974, so that people aren't excluded from jury service just on the grounds that they're having treatment for a mental illness. And it amends the Companies (Model Articles) Regulations 2008 so that a person can continue to be a director of a company even though a court has made an order, on grounds of their mental health, that prevents them from exercising the powers or rights they would otherwise have.

- Secondary legislation:
  - Tribunal directions for Responsible Clinician's reports for tribunal hearings;
  - Amendments to Tribunal rules:
    - to make the medical examination discretionary (except in section 2 cases, where there is to be no change);
    - to allow any member of the tribunal to view the medical records (rather than just the Medical Member);
    - to require either a medical examination or a finding that one is unnecessary or not practicable before a Tribunal can proceed in the patient's absence;
    - Secretary of State's 2014 instructions with respect to the exercise of approval functions for section 12 and Approved Clinician approval.

Other changes are due to court judgments. The most difficult areas are the interface between the Mental Health Act and the Mental Capacity Act and the continuing dilemma of what, exactly, amounts to deprivation of liberty.

There is also revised guidance in relation to applying for section 12 and/or Approved Clinician approval.

Preface to the Fourth Edition

Since publication of the third edition, the Care Act 2014 has amended section 117 of the Mental Health Act 1983 (MHA). It now includes a definition of aftercare services: such services (a) meet a need arising from or related to a person's mental disorder; and (b) reduce the risk of deterioration of a person's mental condition (and, accordingly, reduce the risk of the person requiring re-admission to hospital for treatment for the disorder). This replaces the previous judicial interpretation. Which local authority has to pay for a person's section 117 aftercare has also been changed. It is now the authority in which the person was 'ordinarily resident' immediately before detention.

There is a revised MHA Code of Practice and a revised Reference Guide. Leaving aside changes required because of amendments to the MHA and other new statutes since the previous Code was written (e.g. the Health and Social Care Act 2012 and the Care Act 2014), the tone of the new Code is very different from its predecessor. There is much more emphasis on human rights and equality (including the Human Rights Act and other relevant legislation) with significant changes to the Principles underpinning use of the MHA.

As always, there is a great deal of new case law.

It may also be noticed that Nick Brindle has joined Tony Zigmond as author. T. Z. retired from clinical practice some years ago and, given that this is a clinician's guide, he decided that a well-informed practising psychiatrist was a necessary addition to the authorship. This is T. Z.'s final edition of *A Clinician's Brief Guide to the Mental Health Act*, but he is sure that it will continue to be updated as necessary. He is extremely grateful to all those who have encouraged him, praised and, most importantly, bought the book.

Preface to the Fifth Edition

The law, perhaps even more than clinical medicine, is in a state of unremitting development and elaboration. New statutes are passed and changes to the interpretation of existing Acts may modify or transform what was previously accepted practice. It can be difficult for clinicians, and others, to keep up to date. For example, since publication of the fourth edition:

- There have been many noteworthy cases relating to a person's Article 5 rights under the European Convention on Human Rights, i.e. the right to liberty and security. These cases are important in many clinical settings because they affect how the right is to be interpreted and the complex rules for when and how a patient may be deprived of their liberty.
- Of relevance to clinical practice is that there are now different decisions for which capacity may need to be assessed in relation to a patient's application to, and representation at, the Tribunal. The Tribunal is the legal forum which determines whether grounds for detention under the Mental Health Act exist.

These and other changes due to court judgments are discussed. England and Wales are also on the cusp of important legal and practice changes as a result of the Mental Capacity Amendment Act 2019, which received royal assent in May 2019. This will introduce a new process for authorising deprivations of liberty (the Liberty Protection Safeguards), replacing the Deprivation of Liberty Safeguards introduced in 2008. In the final chapter, we briefly discuss proposals to reform the Mental Health Act to address issues relating to the rising rates of people being detained and the disproportionate number of people from black and minority ethnic groups detained under the Mental Health Act. Some readers may notice that T. Z. is an author despite the statement in the preface to the fourth edition that he wouldn't be. This was at the request of N. B.

List of Abbreviations

A&E	Accident and Emergency
AC	Approved Clinician
AMCP	Approved Mental Capacity Professional
AMHP	Approved Mental Health Professional
AWOL	absent without leave
BIA	Best Interests Assessor
BNF	British National Formulary
CAMHS	Child and Adolescent Mental Health Services
CCG	Clinical Commissioning Group
CQC	Care Quality Commission
CTO	Community Treatment Order
DHSC	Department of Health and Social Care
DoL	Deprivation of Liberty
DoLS	Deprivation of Liberty Safeguards
DSM	Diagnostic and Statistical Manual of Mental Disorders
ECHR	European Convention on Human Rights
ECT	electroconvulsive therapy
ECtHR	European Court of Human Rights
FTT	First-Tier Tribunal (Mental Health)
GMC	General Medical Council
GPwSI	General Practitioner with a Special Interest
HM	Hospital Manager
HRA	Human Rights Act 1998
ICD	International Classification of Diseases
IJ	Inherent jurisdiction
IMCA	Independent Mental Capacity Advocate
IMHA	Independent Mental Health Advocate
LPS	Liberty Protection Safeguards
MCA	Mental Capacity Act 2005
MHA	Mental Health Act 1983
MM	Medical Member of the Tribunal (see below)
ND	Nominated Deputy
NP	Nominated Person
NR	Nearest Relative
RB	Responsible Body
RC	Responsible Clinician
RMP	Registered Medical Practitioner
SCT	Supervised Community Treatment
SOAD	Second Opinion Appointed Doctor
FTT	First-Tier Tribunal (Mental Health)

Setting the Scene, Statutory Law and the Common Law

The law, like medicine, is full of 'ifs' and 'buts', with 'not yet determined' in place of the medical 'not yet known'. In that it is 'man-made' it is simpler than medicine, but it has the added complication that it does not remain static, being amended by Parliament and the courts as the attitudes of society change. Although some questions have a clear answer, a 'right' or 'wrong' or 'lawful' or 'unlawful', most do not. Rarely, this is because there is no law. More commonly, it is because the law could be interpreted in several ways and, as yet, there hasn't been a relevant court case or, as will be seen, there have been many cases with different judges interpreting the law in different ways.

It is also important to recognise that our clinical decisions are influenced by many factors other than the law. The first, and most important, is clinical need, combined with the expressed wishes of the patient. Other 'controls' include:

- Codes of Practice, such as those relating to the Mental Health Act 1983,[1, 2] the Mental Capacity Act 2005[3] and the Mental Capacity Act Deprivation of Liberty Safeguards,[4] and the Mental Health Act Reference Guide;[5]
- government circulars and directives, such as the Care Programme Approach and mandatory homicide inquiries;
- the General Medical Council and other regulatory bodies;
- terms and conditions of employment;
- availability of resources;
- public opinion and the media;
- fear of being sued or making a career-limiting mistake.

> **Note**
>
> Although England and Wales have their own Codes of Practice in relation to the Mental Health Act, the Codes pertaining to the Mental Capacity Act and the Deprivation of Liberty Safeguards are the same for England and Wales. A new Mental Capacity Act Code of Practice including, among other things, the Liberty Protection Safeguards, is imminent at the time of writing.

What Is Meant by 'the Law'?

Statute (Parliamentary) Law

Statute laws are passed by Parliament and called Acts of Parliament. There have been many Acts relating to the care, control and treatment of mentally disordered people, dating back as far as 1324 (a sort of early guardianship order which permitted the King to take over the estate of people with a learning/intellectual disability). Over the past 300 years, more than 40 important (at the time) Acts have been passed in this area. Thankfully, only a few are relevant today.

Unlike most other countries, the United Kingdom (UK) does not have a written constitution, but instead has an accumulation of various statutes, conventions, judicial decisions and treaties. Parliamentary sovereignty is a defining principle of the UK Constitution and as such statute law can only be changed by Parliament. However, when the UK was a member state of the European Union (EU), Parliament then accepted that in the areas of law governed by the EU, the latter's laws prevailed over UK law. In effect, there was a contract by which the UK, as a sovereign state, agreed to some limitations on sovereignty. Parliament nonetheless remains the ultimate authority given one Parliament cannot bind another. Therefore, following the UK's withdrawal from the European Union, the European Communities Act 1972 was repealed thereby European Union law no longer has supremacy over legislation passed by the UK Parliament and rulings made by UK courts. The only remaining 'higher authority' comes from the Council of Europe, distinct from the European Union, and which drew up the European Convention on Human Rights (ECHR). If a current law is judged by the European Court of Human Rights (ECtHR) to clash with this Convention, then Parliament is obliged to change the law. The European Court of Human Rights cannot, by itself, change UK law.

Before being passed by Parliament, Acts are called Bills and their paragraphs are called 'clauses'. Following Royal Assent, at the end of the Parliamentary process, when the Bill becomes an Act, paragraphs are called 'sections' (usually followed by a numeric code, e.g. section 5(2) – which, as an aside, in the Mental Health Act 1983 (MHA) authorises hospital authorities to stop an informally admitted (voluntary) patient from leaving hospital). The equivalent in the European Court of Human Rights are called 'articles'.

Acts of Parliament are also referred to as primary legislation. Scotland and Northern Ireland have their own primary legislation passed by their own legislatures (a Parliament in Scotland and an Assembly in Northern Ireland). Until 2020, Wales had an Assembly with more limited powers (see Appendix 1, section A1.1). Primary legislation passed by the Welsh Assembly was called a Measure. Wales now has a Parliament, not an Assembly, and its laws are Acts, not measures. When this book refers to Acts, or primary legislation, it is usually relevant in both England and Wales, but not in Scotland or Northern Ireland.

Note

Where the legislation and personnel differ between England and Wales, the main text of this book gives the English version. The important equivalents for Wales are given in Appendix 1. In addition, for Wales:

- for Secretary of State for Health read Welsh Ministers;
- for Clinical Commissioning Group read Local Health Board;
- for Care Quality Commission read Healthcare Inspectorate Wales;
- for Mental Health Tribunal read Mental Health Review Tribunal for Wales.

Some Acts, such as most of the Mental Capacity Act, are very easy to read. Others, such as the consent to treatment provisions for patients on Community Treatment Orders in the Mental Health Act, can, in part, be very hard going indeed.

Acts of relevance to mental health professionals in England and Wales are:

- the Mental Health Act 1983 (MHA);
- the Human Rights Act 1998 (HRA);
- the Mental Capacity Act 2005 (MCA).

Secondary Legislation, Including Statutory Instruments

These are also 'the law' and must be obeyed, but they are determined by government rather than Parliament (within a defined scope and under discretion granted by Parliament in the relevant Act). England and Wales have differing secondary legislation. The relevant text of this book relates to the secondary legislation in England, but, to assist readers, some guidance relating to Wales is included.

Examples of secondary legislation regarding healthcare include:

- the rules for being appointed as an Approved Clinician;[6]
- rules governing the functioning of First-Tier Tribunals (Mental Health);[7] the official term for Mental Health Tribunals (see Chapter 4, 'Who's Involved?').

The Role of the Courts, Common Law and Statutory Interpretation

'Common law' is judge-made law ('common sense under a wig' was how Lord Donaldson expressed it[8]). Before the establishment of common law, England and Wales had feudal laws, trial by ordeal (e.g. walking over hot coals) and Church law. It is called common law because it is common to all England. It is a body of law made up entirely of principles developed organically from individual cases on a case-by-case basis.

To return to Lord Donaldson:[9]

> The common law is the great safety net which lies behind all statute law and is capable of filling gaps left by that law, if and insofar as those gaps have to be filled in the interests of society as a whole. This process of using the common law to fill gaps is one of the most important duties of the judges. It is not a legislative function or process – that is an alternative solution the initiation of which is the sole prerogative of Parliament. It is an essentially judicial process and, as such, it has to be undertaken in accordance with principle.

Judges also interpret the statutes passed by Parliament and make rulings on these. English and Welsh law operates through a system of precedents (or binding rules). Courts are in a hierarchy of authority, with the Supreme Court at the apex, the Court of Appeal below it and the High Court below that. Once a higher court makes a ruling, the courts lower in the hierarchy are bound to apply it unless they can find a reason why it is not applicable in the particular circumstances of the case in front of them. Therefore, if the Supreme Court has made a decision, all the lower courts and tribunals must follow it until the Supreme Court makes a new, different ruling.

Court judgments lay down new rules or apply existing rules from previous cases. The rule laid down in the case is called the *ratio decidendi* and remarks that relate to it or explain it further are called *obiter dicta*. The rules may be quite specific to the circumstances of the particular case and therefore applicable only in very similar circumstances, or they may be more easily generalised to other situations. Problems in deciding just what the law is include:

- ensuring that your case's circumstances are similar to the one about which the judge has pronounced; this is particularly important when there have been a number of apparently similar cases but the different judges have given very different interpretations (e.g. a significant problem in relation to defining 'deprivation of liberty');

• being confident that there isn't a later case that gives a different interpretation (to exactly the same set of circumstances or wording in an Act) or that a court higher up the hierarchy has not made a different decision;

• clarifying that the judge's statements were not *obiter dicta*, meaning that the judge does not wish them to be used as a 'precedent' (i.e. a decision that must be followed in future by lower courts).

You may come across the term 'inherent jurisdiction' (IJ) of the High Court. This is the right of a court to hear any matter it believes it should hear unless there is a statute or rule which prevents it from doing so. For example, before the MCA, who decided whether or not a doctor could give medical treatment to a patient who lacked the capacity to consent to it? The inherent jurisdiction of the High Court gave the court the right to make that decision. That jurisdiction ceased once there was relevant statute law, in this case the MCA. The inherent jurisdiction may still be used when the person has capacity but is vulnerable or, for example, in a mental health setting when it appears that neither the MHA nor the MCA apply. We will discuss cases in which the inherent jurisdiction has been applied in subsequent chapters.

Yet another role of the High Court is that of Judicial Review. Its purpose is to keep a check on any public body carrying out a public decision-making function. If you believe that a public body has made a decision without giving proper regard to all the issues, e.g. you are refused a medical treatment on the National Health Service (NHS), then you can ask the court to order the body to review its decision. The court will determine whether the decision made was undertaken illegally, irrationally or unreasonably. Judicial Reviews are only available if there is no other right of Appeal against a decision. An example in the MHA is that the only way to challenge the decision of the Mental Health Tribunal used to be by Judicial Review. This changed in 2008 when the Upper Tribunal was established, giving a means to appeal a Tribunal decision and so removing the right to Judicial Review. However, there continues to be no other means of appealing against the decision of a Second Opinion Appointed Doctor (SOAD) and so the Judicial Review option remains. An example is that of Mr W, where the court ruled that a SOAD is required to give reasons for their decision to endorse a treatment plan (section 58 of the MHA).[10]

The following examples are just to illustrate how judge-made law works. How it all fits together is explained in later chapters.

Resolving an Argument

Question   Can an informal (i.e. not detained under the MHA) mentally ill person who retains full decision-making capacity be restrained (other than in the same circumstances as anyone can be – to prevent the commission of a crime)?

Answer   In very limited circumstances: 'This power [common law power to restrain] is confined to imposing temporary restraint on a lunatic who has run amok and is a manifest danger to himself or to others – a state of affairs as obvious to a layman as to a doctor'.[11]

Question   If a person is symptom free, but only because they are taking medication for a disorder, can they still be described as suffering from the disorder?

Answer   Yes: 'It is said, and said with much force, that so long as it is necessary for a person to be under treatment for a disease or disability, then that person must be held to be suffering from that disease or disability. In my judgement that is in general right'.[12]

Interpretation of the MHA

Question The MHA authorises treatment of mental disorder. But what is treatment for mental disorder as opposed to treatment for physical disorder? If a patient suffers from depression secondary to thyroid disease, would treatment of the thyroid problem be considered treatment for mental disorder? The particular question, in the court case *B v. Croydon Health Authority*,[13] related to whether or not nasogastric feeding of a patient with borderline personality disorder and secondary anorexia, who was refusing to eat as an act of self-harm, was treatment for the mental disorder.

Answer   The court said that a range of acts ancillary to the core treatment that the patient is receiving fall within the term 'medical treatment' as defined in section 145 of the MHA. Treatment may be considered to be ancillary to the core treatment if it is nursing and care concurrent with the 'core treatment or as a necessary prerequisite to such treatment or to prevent the patient from causing harm to himself or to alleviate the consequences of the disorder'. This judgment is discussed further in Chapter 8.

Care is required when looking at the way judges interpret the statute. Subsequent cases may lead to differing interpretation even though the wording in the Act remains unaltered.

Question Can section 3 of the MHA be renewed while the patient is on long-term leave from the hospital? Until 1986, a small number of patients detained under section 3 would be sent on long-term leave from hospital. Just before their section expired, they would be readmitted to hospital overnight, their section 3 would be renewed and then they would be sent back on leave.

Answer   No, it can't. In the case of *R. v. Hallstrom*,[14] the judge pointed out that when detaining a patient under section 3, or renewing the detention, the doctor was saying that the patient needed to be detained in hospital for treatment of their mental disorder. How, then, could they be deemed well enough to be sent on leave again straight away?

Leave of absence may only be revoked and the patient recalled to hospital when it is necessary in the interests of his health or safety or for the protection of other persons that he again becomes an in-patient. It is therefore unlawful to recall a patient to hospital when the intention is merely to prevent him from being continuously on leave of absence for six months and therefore ceasing to be liable to be recalled to hospital.[15]

The practice of recalling and renewing the section ended in 1986.

The law, and so practice, changed in 1999 following the case of *B v. Barking, Havering and Brentwood Community Healthcare NHS Trust*.[16] A patient detained under section 3 was gradually being discharged from hospital. During the first week she spent one night at home and six in hospital. The next week she spent two nights at home, with the plan to increase the nights at home each week.

She had got as far as five nights at home and two in hospital when the section 3 was renewed. And so the correct answer to the question became:

Answer   Yes, it can if the patient is at times an in-patient. The court decided that renewal was lawful because the patient's care plan included a requirement that she spend time in hospital.

This continued to be the law until 2002. A patient was detained under section 3 but was on long-term leave.[17] She was required to attend the hospital twice a week, one day for occupational therapy and another day to see the consultant psychiatrist in the ward round. In terms of our question, the correct answer changed again:

Answer The judge said this was lawful, despite her not needing to be detained 'in hospital', because, in his opinion (and it is his opinion that counts), there is no distinction between 'in hospital' and 'at hospital'. What mattered was that 'the treatment' was to take place in/at hospital. In the first edition of this book the question was asked: 'Would a requirement for the patient to attend one day a week, or one day a fortnight be enough? We don't know. Perhaps we need another case', and continued in the following way: 'However, the use of extended leave has, perhaps, been superseded by the option of Community Treatment Orders'. Although the last comment may be true, we do have two further cases that appear to loosen the requirement to be 'in' or 'at' hospital to justify the ongoing necessity for section 3.

The first of these, the patient, detained for many weeks under section 3, was granted section 17 leave with the condition that he attend the out-patient clinic every 2 weeks. He appealed to the Tribunal (unsuccessfully), and then to the Upper Tribunal,[18] that he should be discharged because his treatment plan didn't require him to be in hospital. He was again unsuccessful. As the judge said, 'It is important to note that section 145 of the 1983 Act defines "hospital" so that it includes "any health service hospital within the meaning of the National Health Service Act 2006", which in turn includes "any institution for the reception and treatment of persons suffering from illness" and any "clinics, dispensaries and out-patient departments maintained in connection with any such ... institution"'. And so once every 2 weeks, to an out-patient clinic, is enough.

The second relates to a gentleman, Mr L, who was living outside hospital on section 17 leave (in a care home) and required to attend hospital for fortnightly psychology sessions and a monthly ward round.[19] After an unsuccessful appeal to the Mental Health Tribunal, he challenged the decision. The grounds were that almost all the treatment was being delivered in the community, so he no longer justified being subject to section 3. The Upper Tribunal disagreed and confirmed that the tribunal had properly applied the correct legal test. Medical treatment includes rehabilitation under medical supervision, which meant that the section 17 leave and the rehabilitation provided outside hospital, both of which operated under medical supervision, were themselves part of his treatment plan.

This demonstrates one of the problems for clinicians. The relevant wording of the Act hasn't changed at all. And yet we've gone from no renewal of detention unless the patient needs to be in hospital, to legal renewal while the patient is on leave and the only requirement is to attend an out-patient clinic and/or a ward round.

Notes

- Common law cannot be used if there is a statutory alternative.
- Most questions have not yet been answered.

Finally, although not law in the sense used above, the United Kingdom is a signatory to the UN Convention on the Rights of Persons with Disabilities (UNCRPD) 2006. The convention obligates states to (among many other things):

- adopt all appropriate legislative, administrative and other measures for the implementation of the rights recognised in the present Convention;
- take all appropriate measures, including legislation, to modify or abolish existing laws, regulations, customs and practices that constitute discrimination against persons with disabilities.

To explain this further, in September 2014, the UN Office of the High Commissioner for Human Rights issued the following statement concerning Article 14 of the UNCRPD:[20]

> Liberty and security of the person is one of the most precious rights to which everyone is entitled. In particular, all persons with disabilities, and especially persons with mental disabilities or psychosocial disabilities are entitled to liberty pursuant to article 14 of the Convention.
>
> Ever since the CRPD committee began reviewing state party reports at its fifth session in April 2011, the Committee has systematically called to the attention of states party the need to correctly enforce this Convention right. The jurisprudence of the Committee on article 14 can be more easily comprehended by unpacking its various elements as follows:
>
> 1. The absolute prohibition of detention on the basis of disability. There are still practices in which state parties allow for the deprivation of liberty on the grounds of actual or perceived disability. In this regard the Committee has established that article 14 does not permit any exceptions whereby persons may be detained on the grounds of their actual or perceived disability. However, legislation of several states party, including mental health laws, still provide instances in which persons may be detained on the grounds of their actual or perceived disability, provided there are other reasons for their detention, including that they are dangerous to themselves or to others. This practice is incompatible with article 14 as interpreted by the jurisprudence of the CRPD committee.
>
> 2. ... The involuntary detention of persons with disabilities based on presumptions of risk or dangerousness tied to disability labels its contrary to the right to liberty. For example, it is wrong to detain someone just because they are diagnosed with paranoid schizophrenia.

In October 2017,[21] the United Nations published the report of its last examination of how well the United Kingdom is implementing the treaty. One of the recommendations was to 'abolish all forms of substituted decision-making concerning all spheres and areas of life by reviewing and adopting new legislation in accordance with the Convention to initiate new policies in both mental capacity and mental health laws'. The UK Government strongly disagreed with the conclusions reached[22] and at the time of writing and, we suspect, for the foreseeable future, the United Kingdom will not comply. In fairness, we should add that we are not aware of any country which has law compliant with the UNCRPD.

On a personal note, we must mention that one of us (T. Z.), as long ago as 1998, wrote that the Royal College of Psychiatrists 'should consider campaigning for the abolition of a distinct mental health act which only adds to the stigmatisation of the mentally ill'.[23]

To conclude, we will encounter further examples of how decisions in the court have resolved issues that have vexed both practitioners and the courts, with greater or lesser impact. For example, what constitutes a deprivation of a person's liberty? What constitutes treatment for mental disorder? Ultimately, clinicians need to be vigilant about whether the court's intervention is required because there is dispute or a specific legal requirement in relation to their patient. The circumstances may arise when it is necessary to obtain authority from a court as the lawfulness of a treatment (either to be given or withdrawn) when a patient refuses, lacks capacity or there is a difference of opinion regarding best interests. In other cases, a judgment from the court may protect a clinician from claims that he or she has acted unlawfully. The court is also there to safeguard the welfare of the patient.

The Human Rights Act in Clinical Practice

European Law

Understanding European institutions isn't easy or, thankfully, necessary here. Our concern is with the European Convention on Human Rights and Fundamental Freedoms. This was adopted by the Council of Europe (a group of 42 states) in 1951. The United Kingdom was one of the first signatories to the Convention. Although prior to 2000, when the Human Rights Act 1998 (HRA) came into force, 'public authorities' (the term used to describe 'the State') and private institutions providing public functions were supposedly obliged to comply with the European Convention of Human Rights, it was difficult in practice for an aggrieved person to obtain a judgment because they needed to exhaust all domestic legal remedies before they could appeal to the European Convention of Human Rights. The Human Rights Act changed this. Parliament is required to ensure that its laws are compliant with the European Convention of Human Rights, and courts and other public authorities are required to interpret Acts in line with the Convention as far as possible. European Court of Human Rights judgments are applicable in UK courts (although not binding).

There have been many national and international milestones that have shaped the concept of human rights in Britain over the last 800 years. The Magna Carta (1215) acknowledged for the first time that subjects of the Crown had legal rights and that laws could also apply to monarchs. The Habeus Corpus Act (1679) developed the right of a detained person to go before a judge to determine whether the detention was legal. The English Bill of Rights (1689) prohibited the 'infliction of cruel and unusual punishments'. The many treaties and laws inspired by and passed in the years following the Universal Declaration of Human Rights (1948) have had the purpose of tackling discrimination and promoting rights and freedoms. Most recently, the Equality Act (2010) brought together more than 116 separate pieces of legislation into a single Act to provide a legal framework to protect the rights of individuals and advance equality.

The Human Rights Act 1998

The Human Rights Act incorporated the European Conventyion of Human Rights into UK law. In clinical practice, references to the Human Rights Act and to the European Conventyion of Human Rights are interchangeable. The purpose of the Convention is to ensure that governments behave with a proper regard for human rights (it followed the atrocities of the Second World War). It does not apply directly to private companies or citizens unless they are carrying out public functions in the place of the government. It is for governments to legislate to make private bodies and citizens behave properly. It is unlawful for a public authority (the government or its agents) to act incompatibly with the European Conventyion of Human Rights. If they do, the Convention allows for a case to be brought in a UK court. Clinicians, when treating a National Health Service (NHS) patient or a private patient on behalf of the State, act as public authorities. They do not do so when treating paying private patients. Private hospitals are public authorities when providing services to NHS-funded patients. We must keep the European Convention of Human Rights in mind when carrying out our clinical practice. The Articles of major relevance are the following (that's not to say the others are irrelevant):

- Article 2, the right to life;
- Article 3, the prohibition of torture;
- Article 5, the right to liberty and security;
- Article 6, the right to a fair trial;
- Article 8, the right to respect for private and family life.

The European Convention of Human Rights requires all UK legislation to be interpreted, as far as possible, in accordance with Convention rights. If a UK court decides that it cannot interpret an Act in a way that is compatible with the Convention, it has to make a 'declaration of incompatibility' (between UK law and the European Convention) so that the government can ask Parliament to change the law. This does not override Parliament. The Act remains unaltered until amended by Parliament. Parliament has a fast-track method for amending Acts under such circumstances.

Example

The first declaration of incompatibility, after the Human Rights Act came into force, related to the Mental Health Act 1983. When a patient appealed to a Mental Health Review Tribunal (as the Tribunal was then called) against their detention, the burden of proof was on the patient to prove that criteria justifying detention no longer existed. This was declared incompatible with Article 5 of the European Convention of Human Rights , which requires the detaining authority to prove that a person is of unsound mind if they are to be detained or continue to be detained. A 'remedial order'[1] reversed the burden of proof so it is now up to the hospital to prove that the patient suffers from a mental disorder.

The European Convention of Human Rights is said to be a 'living' document. It is expected that the way courts interpret its Articles will change over time, developing in line with the current mores of society.

There are three categories of rights under the Convention:

- 'absolute' – no excuses (e.g. Article 3);
- 'limited' – there are specific, explicit circumstances, defined in the Article, when it doesn't apply (e.g. Article 5);
- 'qualified' – interference is permitted in a range of circumstances (e.g. Article 8).

One potential difficulty is that one person's rights may compete with another person's. For example, should there be an absolute right to practise one's religion? Clearly not, if to do so involves sacrificing the lives or freedoms of others. Furthermore, some Articles appear to clash and a balance must be struck. For example, Article 2, which puts a positive duty on the State to preserve life, may conflict with Article 8, which requires the State not to interfere in people's lives.

This balance, or tension, between Articles was passionately conveyed by a dissenting judge in a European Convention of Human Rights case where a man (Mr J) killed himself while he was a voluntary in-patient in a Portuguese state-run psychiatric institution.[2] By majority, the judges concluded that the Portuguese authorities had not been in breach of their duties. However, the dissenting judge made the following illustrative statement regarding the emerging trend to more liberal, 'open door', regimes in psychiatric hospitals:

> The right to life prevails over the right to liberty, especially when the psychopathological condition of the individual limits his or her capacity for self-determination. It is nothing but pure hypocrisy to argue that the State should leave vulnerable suicidal inpatients in State-run psychiatric hospitals free to put an end to their lives merely in order to respect their right to freedom.

Indeed, there may be a problem even within an Article. Should, for example, a person with a learning disability who cannot make these decisions for themselves be left with their family (assuming that is the family's wish), or be moved to encourage living an independent life (against the family's wish)? Article 8 is respect for both family and private life and has been used by both sides in support of their argument.

One of the most useful concepts introduced by the European Convention of Human Rights is that of 'proportionality'. This says that any interference with a Convention right must be proportionate to the intended aims (and the aims themselves must be legitimate). How much force can be used in a particular circumstance, e.g. an interference with a person's physical integrity or putting a patient in seclusion, depends on the severity of the threat.

Finally, it is perhaps worth noting that only a public authority, including private bodies when exercising public functions, can be sued under the Human Rights Act and only victims can sue. Identifying the victim may not always be obvious. A patient's daughter successfully sued a hospital when her mother, while detained under the MHA, died by suicide (the hospital had breached Article 2, the patient's right to life, by providing care that was not of the required standard),[3] as did the parents of an informal patient who took her own life while on leave (the case is considered further in the next section on Convention Articles).[4]

The following section looks at specific human rights legislation. In an attempt to limit confusion, only the most relevant Articles are reproduced and discussed.

Convention Articles

Article 2: Right to life

1. Everyone's right to life shall be protected by law. No one shall be deprived of his life intentionally save in the execution of a sentence of a court following his conviction of a crime for which this penalty is provided by law.
2. Deprivation of life shall not be regarded as inflicted in contravention of this article when it results from the use of force which is no more than absolutely necessary:
   a. in defence of any person from unlawful violence;
   b. in order to effect a lawful arrest or to prevent escape of a person lawfully detained;
   c. in action lawfully taken for the purpose of quelling a riot or insurrection.

Article 2 is a positive duty on the State to protect the lives of citizens.[5] It may also be engaged when the individual in question does not die, but relevant failures of the State put that individual's life in jeopardy.[6] The courts, having decided that there is a lower threshold for breaching Article 2 when the patient is detained under the MHA (as is also the case for prisoners),[7] have now extended the reach of the Article to informal psychiatric patients.[8] Standards for hospital policies, training and practice must be high when there is a 'real and immediate risk' of suicide. The Supreme Court has made the point that psychiatric patients who have consented to admission to hospital (informal or voluntary patients) may not be in the same position as physically ill patients who have consented, because the former (a) may have impaired capacity, (b) may be consenting because they fear detention and (c) can be detained under section 5 of the MHA.

The case involved a woman, Ms R, who was admitted because of expressed suicidal thoughts. She agreed to admission and so was admitted informally. After a few days, she requested weekend leave. The consultant met with her and her mother in his ward round and agreed to allow her home for 2 days and a night. Ms R killed herself the next day, while on leave. The court decided that her Article 2 right to life had been breached. In addition to emphasising the importance of a proper assessment and good record-keeping, this case raises the issue of what risk qualifies as 'real and immediate'. The expert witness whose assessment was accepted said that the risk of the patient killing herself 'was approximately 5% on 19 April (after the patient left the hospital), increasing to 10% on 20 April and 20% on 21 April' (another expert put the risk at 70 per cent, but the court rejected this). Leaving aside that this risk assessment has been challenged as much too high,[9] even if accepted a risk of 10 per cent was considered high enough to meet the 'real and immediate' test.

Clinicians will acknowledge the challenges of accurate suicide prediction. However, in order to establish whether the authorities knew, or ought to have known, that the life of a particular individual was subject to a 'real and immediate risk', the European Court has taken into account a number of factors (summarised in the Portuguese case referred to above[10]), including:

- whether the person had a history of mental health problems;
- the gravity of the mental condition;
- previous attempts to commit suicide or self-harm;
- suicidal thoughts or threats; and
- signs of physical or mental distress.

An institution will not have breached Article 2 if it has done everything correctly but there is poor practice or negligence by an individual member of staff. Article 2 also covers the clinician's duty to pass on sensitive information about serious risks to a person or hospital when transferring the care of a mentally disordered patient, and the need to consider the risks to other in-patients (e.g. ensuring an appropriate environment if admitting a very disturbed patient). Other examples include: 'do not attempt cardiopulmonary (DNACPR) orders, withdrawal of life-sustaining/prolonging treatments and arguments about when the State will not fund particular treatments. An interesting example arose in a case about conjoined twins.[11] Separating the twins would result in the immediate death of one twin, but not separating them would lead to the death of both. It was argued that one of the twins was interfering in the right to life of the other.

Article 3: Prohibition of torture

No one shall be subjected to torture or to inhuman or degrading treatment or punishment.

Article 3 is an absolute right. In relation to compulsory psychiatric treatment, before the HRA came into force, it was thought that electroconvulsive therapy (ECT) and seclusion might automatically breach Article 3 – they don't (although their use might breach it in specific cases). The provision of medical assistance to a detained person, against that person's will (by force if necessary) in principle will not be in breach of Article 3, however, '[t]he Court must nevertheless satisfy itself that a medical necessity has been convincingly shown to exist and that procedural guarantees for the decision . . . exist and are complied with'.[12]

In the case of *Herczegfalvy* v. *Austria*,[13] a violent, mentally ill patient on hunger strike complained that he had been forcibly administered food and antipsychotics, isolated and attached to a security bed with handcuffs. The European Court of Human Rights held that 'as a general rule a measure which is a therapeutic necessity cannot be regarded as inhuman or degrading'. On a more cautionary note, the court also said 'the position of inferiority and powerlessness which is typical of patients confined in psychiatric hospitals calls for increased vigilance when reviewing compliance with the Convention'.

Based on this case, the threshold to breach Article 3 seems to be set high. Nonetheless, it is of course important to be mindful of the impact coercive treatment may have on your patient. An example is that concerning the treatment of Mr K, a 55-year-old man with autism spectrum disorder.[14] He was detained under section 48 of the MHA and was refusing to eat. The judge concluded that while force feeding was capable of being treatment for the manifestation of his mental disorder, given Mr K's strength of feelings against the intervention, 'if it came to that stage close consideration would necessarily have to be given to the terms of article 3 ECHR and the case law such as Herczegfalvy v Austria [1993] 15 EHRR 437 and the test of medical necessity'.

Neglect of a detained patient that leads to death[15] may also be a breach of Article 3 (rather than Article 2). Article 3 may also be engaged when detaining patients suffering from acute mental-health problems in a place which is entirely ill-adapted to their circumstances. Conditions inside a detainee's (Mr S) cell quickly deteriorated while waiting for a transfer from a police custody to a medium-secure facility that was delayed. The European Court of Human Rights in this case found 'that the conditions which the applicant was required to endure were an affront to human dignity and reached the threshold of degrading treatment for the purposes of Article 3'.[16]

Article 5: Right to liberty and security of person

1   Everyone has the right to liberty and security of person. No one shall be deprived of his liberty save in the following cases and in accordance with a procedure prescribed by law:

   a. the lawful detention of a person after conviction by a competent court;
   b. the lawful arrest or detention of a person for non-compliance with the lawful order of a court or in order to secure the fulfilment of any obligation prescribed by law;
   c. the lawful arrest or detention of a person effected for the purpose of bringing him before the competent legal authority on reasonable suspicion of having committed an offence or when it is reasonably considered necessary to prevent his committing an offence or fleeing after having done so;
   d. the detention of a minor by lawful order for the purpose of educational supervision or his lawful detention for the purpose of bringing him before the competent legal authority;

e. the lawful detention of persons for the prevention of the spreading of infectious diseases, of persons of unsound mind, alcoholics or drug addicts, or vagrants;

f. the lawful arrest or detention of a person to prevent his effecting an unauthorised entry into the country or of a person against whom action is being taken with a view to deportation or extradition.

2. Everyone who is arrested shall be informed promptly, in a language which he understands, of the reasons for his arrest and of any charge against him.

3. Everyone arrested or detained in accordance with the provisions of paragraph 1c. of this Article shall be brought promptly before a judge or other officer authorised by law to exercise judicial power and shall be entitled to trial within a reasonable time or to release pending trial. Release may be conditioned by guarantees to appear for trial.

4. Everyone who is deprived of his liberty by arrest or detention shall be entitled to take proceedings by which the lawfulness of his detention shall be decided speedily by a court and his release ordered if the detention is not lawful.

5. Everyone who has been the victim of arrest or detention in contravention of the provisions of this Article shall have an enforceable right to compensation.

Article 5 is central to issues relating to the MHA and detained patients. There are a number of important points to consider.

'No one shall be deprived of his liberty save in the following cases and in accordance with a procedure prescribed by law' (paragraph 1): this is not an issue in relation to patients detained under the MHA because the MHA is a 'procedure prescribed by law'.

It is, nonetheless, worth considering a little further. What is meant by 'deprived of his liberty'? While the law has been clarified (see below) it often remains difficult to determine in individual cases. In the case known as *Bournewood* (the name of the Trust that managed the hospital), the European Court of Human Rights decided that the patient, Mr L, was deprived of his liberty. He suffered from autism and a learning disability,[17] and he was admitted to hospital having displayed disturbed behaviour at his day centre. He was not capable of consenting or otherwise to his admission to hospital, but he was compliant with it. He did not try to leave the hospital, but would have been stopped had he done so. The ward door was not locked. Mr L's (paid) carers wanted him home. They were not permitted to visit lest Mr L follow them out of the hospital when they left. Nor were they permitted to speak to him on the phone.

The European Court recognised that deprivation of liberty, as opposed to restricting a person's liberty, 'is merely one of degree or intensity and not one of nature or substance' and 'to determine whether there has been a deprivation of liberty, the starting-point must be the specific situation of the individual concerned and account must be taken of a whole range of factors arising in a particular case such as the type, duration, effects and manner of implementation of the measure in question'.[18]

Given that (a) the staff had 'exercised complete and effective control' over Mr L and (b) although he had not tried to leave the ward, had he tried he would have been prevented from doing so, being restrained if necessary, the European Court decided Mr L was deprived of his liberty.

In the case of Mr L, the European Court then turned to the second part of paragraph 1 in Article 5 – 'in accordance with a procedure prescribed by law'. Mr L had been kept in hospital 'under the common law doctrine of necessity'.[19] In other words, there was no 'procedure prescribed by law'. This also meant he was not able 'to take proceedings by which the lawfulness of his detention shall be decided speedily by a court' (another requirement of Article 5, at paragraph 4).

It is not often that such complete control is taken of patients (stopping their visitors, telephone calls and so on) and so the number of deprivations of liberty, apart from patients detained under the MHA, was thought to be small. What is meant by 'deprivation of liberty' is discussed further in Chapter 3.

It is salutary to remember how Mr L finally got his freedom. He was kept in hospital under common law for many months. When it was first decided (by the Court of Appeal) that this was unlawful, he was detained under the MHA. He appealed against detention and was discharged from his section by the Hospital Managers. Detention under the MHA can be liberating!

Central to the MHA is paragraph 1(e) of Article 5, which allows 'the lawful detention of persons for the prevention of the spreading of infectious diseases, of persons of unsound mind, alcoholics or drug addicts, or vagrants'. What is meant by unsound mind and who decides that a person is so suffering? In a pivotal case, *Winterwerp* v. *The Netherlands*,[20] the European Court of Human Rights said:

> A person cannot be detained as being of unsound mind unless he or she is reliably shown to be so as demonstrated by objective medical expertise and the nature or degree of his or her mental disorder is such as to justify the deprivation of liberty. The detention ceases to be valid when the relevant mental disorder disappears or ceases to be such as justifies the deprivation of liberty.

This is important because it means that a detained patient's mental state must be kept under constant review by the clinician responsible for their care and the patient must be discharged from detention under the MHA if they are deemed no longer to be suffering from any mental disorder (this applies even if the patient is in a maximum-security hospital and thought to be dangerous).

Who can provide 'objective medical expertise' is discussed in Chapter 5 in the section titled 'Section 20 – Duration of Authority'.

In a previous edition of this book, paragraphs 3 and 4 of Article 5 were mentioned as follows:

> ... it can be difficult to follow the wording but what these paragraphs say is that if someone is arrested, or detained, in relation to a crime (suspected of or fleeing from), then they must be brought before a court. If they are arrested or detained for any other reason, because of their mental health for example, they have the right to a court hearing – but it is up to them to request one. It has been argued that this means that severely disabled patients, who may not understand their rights and so do not appeal, are disadvantaged. For them, the 'right to appeal' isn't a real right. Whether or not this disadvantage is sufficiently ameliorated by the duty of the Hospital Managers to refer patients to the Tribunal at defined intervals, if the patient hasn't already appealed, is arguable. You may consider it unethical that a patient who isn't well enough to ask for an appeal won't get one, but it isn't a breach of their human rights as defined by the European Convention on Human Rights.[21]

The case that we had in mind concerned a patient with Down syndrome. She was initially detained under section 2. Her Nearest Relative, her mother, tried to discharge her (section 23), but the Responsible Medical Officer (now called the Responsible Clinician) issued a barring order (section 25). The Responsible Medical Officer then wished to place the patient on a guardianship order (see Chapter 5, 'Section 7 – Application for Guardianship'), but could not because the mother, as Nearest Relative, objected (a guardianship order cannot go ahead if the Nearest Relative objects).

An application was made to the court to displace the mother as Nearest Relative (see Chapter 5, 'Additional Points'). Under such circumstances, a section 2 continues until 7 days after the court case. During this time, the mother arranged for solicitors to request the Secretary of State to refer the patient to the Tribunal (section 67), which was done. The Tribunal upheld the continuing detention. The case finally reached the European Court of Human Rights.[22] The court said that the patient's inability to appeal while detained under section 2 was a breach of the Human Rights Act and ordered compensation. The lack of a right to appeal while waiting for the displacement hearing wasn't a breach, in that case, because there was a Tribunal, albeit only because the patient had a determined mother, who requested the Secretary of State to order one.

This same logic was applied in the case of Ms K,[23] who was detained under section 3 (rather than section 2 as in the case of Ms H above) and lacked capacity to apply to the First-Tier Tribunal. Her solicitor made an application on her behalf, but the proceedings were struck out when her lack of capacity emerged. She then applied to the Upper Tribunal to review the Tribunal's decision on the basis '. . . that there is a gap in the legislation that fails to provide for patients who lack the capacity to decide to apply to the First-tier Tribunal'. The judge in the Upper Tribunal made the following statement. 'This case is governed by the reasoning in R (H). There is no violation of the patient's Convention rights. An application for the Secretary of State to refer his case could have been made under section 67 and, if that was refused, the patient could have had recourse to judicial review.'

We would like to draw attention to the comment of Mr Justice Peter Jackson in the case of Mr N that 'there is an obligation on the State to ensure that a person deprived of liberty is not only entitled but enabled to have the lawfulness of his detention reviewed speedily by a court'.[24] Reliance on third parties, such as a determined mother, in order to be able to fulfil the right to a Tribunal is not satisfactory. It seems to us that section 2, and perhaps section 3, should now be deemed incompatible with Article 5 of the European Convention because patients who are too ill to appeal have no real right of appeal.

Article 6: Right to a fair trial

1. In the determination of his civil rights and obligations or of any criminal charge against him, everyone is entitled to a fair and public hearing within a reasonable time by an independent and impartial tribunal established by law. Judgment shall be pronounced publicly but the press and public may be excluded from all or part of the trial in the interest of morals, public order or national security in a democratic society, where the interests of juveniles or the protection of the private life of the parties so require, or to the extent strictly necessary in the opinion of the court in special circumstances where publicity would prejudice the interests of justice.
2. Everyone charged with a criminal offence shall be presumed innocent until proved guilty according to law.
3. Everyone charged with a criminal offence has the following minimum rights:
   a. to be informed promptly, in a language which he understands and in detail, of the nature and cause of the accusation against him;
   b. to have adequate time and facilities for the preparation of his defence;
   c. to defend himself in person or through legal assistance of his own choosing or, if he has not sufficient means to pay for legal assistance, to be given it free when the interests of justice so require;

d. to examine or have examined witnesses against him and to obtain the attendance and examination of witnesses on his behalf under the same conditions as witnesses against him;

e. to have the free assistance of an interpreter if he cannot understand or speak the language used in court.

Article 6 is important not only in relation to civil and criminal cases, but also, for example, in tribunals, General Medical Council and other professional body hearings, and employment and disciplinary procedures. A patient detained under the MHA has the right to have a lawyer unless they actively express the choice not to have one. Although the person has a right to know the case against them, that does not mean that everything in the patient's medical record has to be revealed.

Article 8: Right to respect for private and family life

1. Everyone has the right to respect for his private and family life, his home and his correspondence.

2. There shall be no interference by a public authority with the exercise of this right except such as is in accordance with the law and is necessary in a democratic society in the interests of national security, public safety or the economic well-being of the country, for the prevention of disorder or crime, for the protection of health or morals, or for the protection of the rights and freedoms of others.

The notion of private life in Article 8 is broad and covers an individual's right to personal autonomy and to physical integrity. This is a qualified right. It can be overridden, if necessary, on the grounds given. Consequently, patient confidentiality can be overridden in certain circumstances (e.g. in informing the Driver and Vehicle Licensing Agency (DVLA) about a patient you believe may be unfit to drive, or informing the police about a patient who may pose a danger to others). In such situations, the patient's consent to release information should always be sought, if possible. Article 8 was used in a case arguing that it was unlawful to ban smoking in hospitals that are effectively patients' homes and that the patients cannot leave (the maximum-security hospitals). The court decided that the exceptions within Article 8 were met and upheld the smoking ban.[25] Seclusion, restraint, strip-searching, access to medical records, family visiting rights, same-sex accommodation and so on are other issues that come within the bounds of Article 8.

It has been argued that the authority given by the MHA to force treatment on capacitous refusing patients breaches Article 8. The courts have been clear that it does not and that 'section 58 [of the MHA] lawfully authorises medical treatment against the will of a capacitous detained patient'.[26] This matter is discussed further in Chapter 8.

The administration of covert medical treatment (for either physical or mental disorder) in care homes[27] or hospitals[28] is a serious interference with an individual's Article 8 rights. Which is not to say it cannot happen, but in so doing one should adhere to clear policy and processes for: assessing capacity; consultation; considering the individual's best interests; recording the assessments; care planning; and undertaking review.

The MHA Code of Practice draws attention to the importance of Article 8 for people detained under the Act. 'Privacy, safety and dignity are important constituents of a therapeutic environment. Hospital staff should make conscious efforts to respect the privacy and dignity of patients as far as possible, while maintaining safety, including enabling a patient to wash and dress in private, and to send and receive mail, including in electronic formats, without restriction' (paragraph 8.4). While it is usually an offence to interfere with the Royal Mail, there are limited circumstances where incoming or outgoing mail to or from a patient may be restricted. Section 134 of the MHA concerns the correspondence of patients and we discuss this further in Chapter 5.

We cannot overemphasise the importance in clinical practice of Article 8 and can do no better than quote the European Court: 'the Court reiterates that even a minor interference with the physical integrity of an individual must be regarded as an interference with the right to respect for private life under Article 8, if it is carried out against the individual's will'.[29] Every time we force a patient to take medication or have a blood test it is a potential breach of Article 8. Our defence is that it is in the interests of the patient's health. However, as mentioned previously, the force used and the impact of the investigation or treatment must be proportionate to the legitimate aim.

Article 12: Right to marry

Men and women of marriageable age have the right to marry and to found a family, according to the national laws governing the exercise of this right.

Article 9: Freedom of thought, conscience and religion

1. Everyone has the right to freedom of thought, conscience and religion; this right includes freedom to change his religion or belief and freedom, either alone or in community with others and in public or private, to manifest his religion or belief, in worship, teaching, practice and observance.
2. Freedom to manifest one's religion or beliefs shall be subject only to such limitations as are prescribed by law and are necessary in a democratic society in the interests of public safety, for the protection of public order, health or morals, or for the protection of the rights and freedoms of others.

Article 13: Right to an effective remedy

Everyone whose rights and freedoms as set forth in this Convention are violated shall have an effective remedy before a national authority notwithstanding that the violation has been committed by persons acting in an official capacity.

In relation to Article 13, compensation has, for example, been paid to patients when their Tribunal hearing has been significantly delayed and to the family of a detained patient whose right to life was violated when poor standards enabled her to take her own life (e.g. *Savage* v. *South Essex Partnership NHS Foundation Trust*[30]).

Article 14: Prohibition of discrimination

The enjoyment of the rights and freedoms set forth in this Convention shall be secured without discrimination on any ground such as sex, race, colour, language, religion, political or other opinion, national or social origin, association with a national minority, property, birth or other status.

Article 14 does not give a freestanding right to non-discrimination, but requires the exercise of the other rights to be carried out in a non-discriminatory way. So if there is a distinction between the way people with a mental disorder are treated compared with the treatment of those with a physical disorder, the article might apply.

Chapter 3

Capacity: The Mental Capacity Act and Deprivation of Liberty Safeguards

The Starting Point

You are asked to see an adult patient. You advise a medical intervention, be it admission to hospital, medical investigations or treatment. The patient wishes to take your advice and consents. Why did you need the patient's consent? Well, because of the common law.

> A competent patient has an absolute right to refuse to consent to medical treatment for any reason, rational or irrational, or for no reason at all, even when that decision may lead to his or her death.

So said Dame Elizabeth Butler-Sloss in the case of a woman who was being kept alive by a ventilator.[1] The patient wished the machine to be turned off, even though this would lead to her death. Her doctors had refused to turn it off, despite agreeing she had the capacity to make the decision. The judgment followed a long line of similar judgments. The machine was switched off.

But what if we clinicians go ahead and treat the patient anyway? A doctor who uses physical force to treat a patient and who has not obtained the patient's consent 'is guilty of the civil wrong of trespass to a person; he is also guilty of the criminal offence of assault'.[2] We can be prosecuted by the police and sued by the patient, not to mention being reported to our professional licensing body.

Colleagues on section 12 and Approved Clinician courses still often express the view that medical 'necessity' overrides personal autonomy. In a 2014 case, the judge could not have made the legal position clearer:

> The freedom to choose for oneself is a part of what it means to be a human being. For this reason, anyone capable of making decisions has an absolute right to accept or refuse medical treatment, regardless of the wisdom or consequences of the decision. The decision does not have to be justified to anyone. In the absence of consent any invasion of the body will be a criminal assault. The fact that the intervention is well meaning or therapeutic makes no difference.[3]

If the patient is aged 18 years or over, and has the capacity to make the decision, that individual is autonomous and their consent must be sought and refusal accepted. (For minors, see Chapter 10.)

But suppose the patient is unconscious or unable to consent for some other reason? That is, the patient lacks the capacity to consent (or, in the case of minors, has not yet developed the competence to do so). Or the patient does retain decision-making capacity but suffers from a mental disorder (or, at least, you think they do) and you believe there are significant risks to the patient or others if they are left without the treatment they are refusing. At this point, we turn to statutory law, either the Mental Capacity Act 2005 (MCA) or the Mental Health Act 1983 (MHA), depending on the circumstances.

To be sure that a patient's consent is real, the clinician must be open and honest with them about the illness and the treatment, the risks and benefits, and they must explain things in a way that they can understand. Consent isn't real consent if it is obtained under duress or on the basis of incorrect or incomplete information: 'The duty of the doctor is to explain what he intends to do and its implications in the way a careful and responsible doctor in similar circumstances would have done.'[4] Similarly, General Medical Council (GMC) guidance on decision-making and consent states: 'When recommending an option for treatment or care to a patient you must explain your reasons for doing so, and share information about reasonable alternatives, including the option to take no action. You must not put pressure on a patient to accept your advice.'[5]

The Bolam Test

All clinicians should remember the Bolam test:

> [A doctor] is not guilty of negligence if he has acted in accordance with a practice accepted as proper by a responsible body of medical men skilled in that particular art . . . Putting it the other way round, a man is not negligent, if he is acting in accordance with such a practice, merely because there is a body of opinion who would take a contrary view.[6]

What does this mean in practice? Don't be the first to use a new treatment or the last to use an old one. Check out with colleagues what they do. Not everyone has to agree. There may be two (or more) perfectly proper opinions as to the correct approach. But don't take a course with which all your colleagues disagree. Follow guidance where you are able, and if you depart from it, record why you're not following it, be it for clinical or resource reasons.

Bolam has been watered down slightly by the courts. The problem with the Bolam test, from a judge's point of view, is that it makes clinicians the final arbiters, rather than the courts (and, to judges, that would never do).

In *Bolitho* v. *City and Hackney HA*,[7] a judge said:

> 'In the vast majority of cases the fact that distinguished experts in the field are of a particular opinion will demonstrate the reasonableness of that opinion. In particular, where there are questions of assessment of the relative risks and benefits of adopting a particular medical practice, a reasonable view necessarily presupposes that the relative risks and benefits have been weighed by the experts in forming their opinions. But if, in a rare case, it can be demonstrated that the professional opinion is not capable of withstanding logical analysis, the judge is entitled to hold that the body of opinion is not reasonable or responsible'.
>
> I emphasise that in my view it will very seldom be right for a judge to reach the conclusion that views genuinely held by a competent medical expert are unreasonable. The assessment of medical risks and benefits is a matter of clinical judgment which a judge would not normally be able to make without expert evidence. . . . It is only where a judge can be satisfied that the body of expert opinion cannot be logically supported at all that such opinion will not provide the bench mark by reference to which the defendant's conduct falls to be assessed.

In a fairly recent case,[8] the question was whether or not a pregnant woman of short stature and with insulin-dependent diabetes who was expecting a large baby should have been warned of the risk of shoulder dystocia, and potential subsequent harm to the mother and possibly the baby, if she had a vaginal delivery. Shoulder dystocia 'is the prime concern in diabetic pregnancies which proceed to labour'. The obstetrician, having taken the relevant measurements and in line with accepted practice (and supported by expert witnesses during the trial), determined that the mother should not be told. The obstetrician did not tell the mother because the mother would then have opted for a Caesarian section, which, in the view of the obstetrician and given the small risk to mother and baby, was not in the mother's best interests. As one of the expert witnesses said: 'If doctors were to warn women at risk of shoulder dystocia, you would actually make most women simply request Caesarean section.' The birth was traumatic and the baby was born with severe disabilities. The court decided that (a) had the mother been told of the risks she would have opted for a Caesarian section, and (b) had she had a Caesarean section the baby would not have been harmed.

The court made a number of important statements. The relationship between doctor and patient should not be based on medical paternalism, nor should the patient be entirely dependent on information provided by the doctor. The law,

> 'instead of treating patients as placing themselves in the hands of their doctors (and then being prone to sue their doctors in the event of a disappointing outcome), [should treat] them so far as possible as adults who are capable of understanding that medical treatment is uncertain of success and may involve risks, accepting responsibility for the taking of risks affecting their own lives, and living with the consequences of their choices'.

The judgment emphasised the 'patient's entitlement to decide whether or not to incur' any risks and pointed out that the decision 'does not depend exclusively on medical considerations'. The court said that information about investigations, treatment options and relative risks was within the doctor's expertise, but that

> 'it is a *non sequitur* to conclude that the question whether a risk of injury, or the availability of an alternative form of treatment, ought to be discussed with the patient is also a matter of purely professional judgment. ... Responsibility for determining the nature and extent of a person's rights rests with the courts, not with the medical professions.
>
> Furthermore, because the extent to which a doctor may be inclined to discuss risks with a patient is not determined by medical learning or experience, the application of the *Bolam* test to this question is liable to result in the sanctioning of differences in practice which are attributable not to divergent schools of thought in medical science, but merely to divergent attitudes among doctors as to the degree of respect owed to their patients'.

What ensues is a two-stage 'Montgomery test'. First, consider what risks are or should be known to the medical profession and, second, whether the patient should be told of such risks, with reference to the test of 'materiality'. The test of materiality is determined as being whether a reasonable person in the patient's position would be likely to attach significance to the risk, or whether the doctor should reasonably be aware that the particular patient would be likely to attach significance to it. Although a court can tell us we're all wrong, the Bolam test remains not only an excellent safeguard, but also a good way to decide whether one's practice is reasonable.

Just as we must not force treatment on patients under such circumstances, equally the patient cannot force, or require, us to give medical treatment. Clinicians should only offer medical treatment that they believe is in the patient's best interests. As Lord Donaldson said: 'Consent by itself creates no obligation to treat.'[9]

If the patient lacks the capacity to consent, as determined by the MCA tests, then the provisions of the MCA must guide practice (unless the patient is detained under the MHA).

The Mental Capacity Act 2005

This Act may authorise medical treatment if a patient aged 16 or over (other rules apply for minors below 16 years – see Chapter 10) lacks capacity to make the decision. It also empowers all adults, while they have decision-making capacity, to make provision for a time in the future when they have lost it.

The MCA (section 1) starts with a set of principles:

- a presumption of capacity;
- a right for individuals to be supported to make their own decisions;
- a right to make unwise decisions;
- that anything done for or on behalf of people without capacity must be done in their best interests;
- that anything done for or on behalf of people without capacity should be the least restrictive of their rights and freedom of action.

In relation to decision-making capacity:

- Assessments of capacity relate to the decision to be made at the time of the assessment. They are decision and time specific. In other words, one should not describe a person as 'lacking capacity': a person lacks capacity at this time, in relation to this decision.
- A person cannot lack capacity unless they have an impairment of, or a disturbance in the functioning of, the mind or brain (section 2 of the MCA).
- A person lacks capacity if, in addition to the previous point, they are unable to understand the information relevant to the decision, to retain that information, to use or weigh that information as part of the process of making the decision, or to communicate their decision. This is the 'functional' approach to assessing a person's capacity (section 3 of the MCA). The information relevant to a decision includes that relating to the reasonably foreseeable consequences of (a) deciding one way or another and (b) failing to make the decision. If the person 'fails' on any of these, they are said to lack capacity in relation to the decision in question.

There is a burgeoning requirement for assessments of capacity to be completed in clinical settings. Assessments of an individual's decision-making capacity are important judgments required to be made at different points during a person's in-patient psychiatric admission. Examples include the following:

- Following admission, an assessment needs to be made in relation to the person's capacity to consent to admission and treatment for mental disorder.
- For those detained under the MHA, there is a statutory requirement to assess capacity preceding the '3-month rule' under section 58 in relation to medication for mental disorder. Although capacity to consent to admission will need to be assessed *prior to* admission (in order to determine the correct legal basis), the Care Quality Commission will look for evidence of these first two assessments as part of their MHA inspection process.
- Capacity to decide whether to obtain help from an Independent Mental Health Advocate (IMHA) will need to be made and, if lacking, one should make further attempts to explain the role to the patient.
- In relation to the Tribunal, a Practice Direction requires that reports submitted by the Responsible Clinician (RC) contain a 'summary of the patient's current progress, behaviour, capacity and insight'.[10]

- The theme of capacity has emerged as a thread through a number of cases in the Upper Tribunal. The relevance to clinical practice is that there are now different decisions for which capacity may need to be assessed in relation to a patient's application to, and representation at, the Tribunal. These cases provide guidance as to how the clinician should apply the statutory test contained in the MCA. We will discuss this issue further in Chapter 9.

Assessment of decision-making can be complex. It may be affected by a combination of factors that vary between individuals and which depend upon, for example, beliefs and values that in turn are influenced by society, culture and education, together with the predispositions of family and peer groups. Even when cognitive functioning may be compromised, for instance by dementia, a person may still be able to express important deep-rooted values underpinning their decisions. In this context, *supporting decision-making* refers to any process in which an individual is provided with as much support as they need in order for them to either make a decision for themselves or express their will and preferences, within the context of substituted decision-making. It is advisable, therefore, to think not just in terms of the test being set out in sections 2 and 3 of the Act but, rather, sections 1, 2 and 3 with the principles, including how decision-making has been supported, applied at the outset.

Giving proper regard to the 'rights, will and preferences' of the person lacking capacity is one way the courts have provided a CRPD-compliant model of best interests decision-making.[11] It also finds a corollary in the proposed reforms to the MHA in the form of the Advance Choice Document (see Chapter 12).

Having determined that the patient is incapable of making the necessary decision, we must first consider three questions.

1. **Has the patient made an advance statement in relation to this decision?**
   An advance statement is a capacitous person's expressed wishes about treatment which become relevant should the person lose capacity to make the relevant decisions in the future. It turns an incapacitous person into a capacitous one (with regard to the specific decision). As with a capacitous decision, if it is a request for treatment the clinician must give it due consideration, but is not bound by it. If it is an advance refusal of treatment, then the clinician is bound by it.

   - To be applicable, the advance decision must closely mirror the current circumstances.
   - An advance decision does not have to be in writing unless it relates to the withholding or withdrawing of life-sustaining treatment.
   - If it does relate to the withholding or withdrawing of life-sustaining treatment, then it must be in writing, signed and the signing must be witnessed and signed (by any adult). If the person is unable to write or sign (e.g. because they have advanced motor neuron disease), then someone else may sign on their behalf. There must be no doubt that it is the person's expressed wish.[12]
   - The advance decision is nullified if the person has, when capacitous but after making the advance decision, acted in a way that is incompatible with the advance decision.
   - An advance decision is invalid if:
     - the patient has capacity to give or refuse consent to it;
     - the patient has withdrawn the decision at a time when they had capacity to do so;

- the patient has, under a lasting power of attorney (see question 2), created after the advance decision was made, conferred authority on the attorney to give or refuse consent to the treatment to which the advance decision relates;
- treatment to be given is not the treatment specified in the advance decision;
- any circumstances specified in the advance decision are absent;
- there are reasonable grounds for believing that circumstances exist that were not anticipated at the time of the advance decision and that would have affected the decision had the person anticipated them;
- the person has done anything else clearly inconsistent with the advance decision remaining their fixed decision.

- Advance decisions/refusals are about medical treatment. One cannot make an advance decision, for example, to refuse basic care or to refuse to go into a care home.

2. **Has the person given someone else the authority to make treatment decisions for them, i.e. given another adult the lasting power of attorney in relation to health and welfare decisions?**
This would mean that the attorney could consent to, or refuse, treatment as if they were the patient. This excludes decisions relating to the withholding or withdrawing of life-sustaining treatment unless they are specifically included. The lasting power of attorney must be registered with the Office of the Public Guardian.
It should be noted that the attorney's power, like an advance refusal, does not come into force until the donor (i.e. the patient) has lost capacity. This is different from a lasting power of attorney for finance, where the donor and attorney can both make decisions until the donor loses capacity (when only the attorney can).

3. **Has the Court of Protection made a decision or appointed a deputy to make the decision?**
Most commonly, none of these will apply. At this point, we must act in the patient's best interests. To do so we must:
- decide whether the patient is likely to regain capacity;
- encourage the patient to participate in the decision;
- take into account:

  - the patient's past and present wishes and feelings (including advance decisions and advance statements);
  - the patient's beliefs and values, if known, that would be likely to influence their decision if they had capacity;
  - anyone named by the patient as someone to be consulted on the matter in question or on matters of that kind;
  - anyone engaged in caring for the patient or interested in their welfare;
  - any agent of a lasting power of attorney granted by the patient;
  - any deputy appointed for the patient by the court;
  - the Independent Mental Capacity Advocate (if there is one).

- in considering best interests in relation to life-sustaining treatment, not be motivated by a desire to bring about the patient's death.

There are specific circumstances when you must involve an Independent Mental Capacity Advocate:

- when 'serious medical treatment' is provided by the NHS, i.e. in any of the following situations:
  - where there is a fine balance between the benefits and burdens of treatment;
  - where a choice of treatments is finely balanced;
  - where what is proposed is likely to have serious consequences for the patient; or
  - cause serious and prolonged pain or serious distress or side-effects; or
  - result in potentially adverse consequences for the patient (e.g. the withdrawal of artificial nutrition and hydration or of other treatment which, if administered, would prolong life in a patient who is terminally ill); or
  - would have a substantial impact on the patient's future life choices (e.g. interventions for ovarian/prostate cancer or sterilisation).

The MCA Code of Practice gives some examples of potentially serious medical treatment:

- chemotherapy and surgery for certain types of cancer;
- electroconvulsive therapy;
- therapeutic sterilisation;
- major surgery such as open-heart surgery or brain/neurosurgery (this excludes psychosurgery, which is covered by the provisions of section 37 of the MHA, i.e. it requires the consent of a capacitous patient and an MHA second opinion);
- major amputations such as the loss of an arm or leg;
- treatments that will result in permanent loss of hearing or sight;
- withholding/withdrawing of artificial nutrition and hydration;
- termination of pregnancy.

There are some medical interventions that require court decisions:

- organ/bone marrow donation by the patient;
- sterilisation for contraception.

It used to be the case that withholding or withdrawing artificial nutrition or hydration from patients in a persistent vegetative state required a court order. The clear steer now provided by the courts in these cases is that where there is unanimity of view as to outcome from treating clinicians, family members and other interested parties, there is no necessity for the decision to be ratified by the courts.

Sections 30 to 34 of the MCA set out detailed rules governing research involving a person who lacks the capacity to consent.

An Independent Mental Capacity Advocate may also be required:

- if an NHS body intends to arrange for a patient to be accommodated:
  - in a hospital for a period likely to exceed 28 days; or
  - in a care home for a period likely to 8 weeks;

- or if an NHS body intends to move the patient between such accommodation (for more than 8 weeks)
- if there are disputes as to the patient's best interests between, for example, family members.

It should be noted that an Independent Mental Capacity Advocate is not required if the moves or treatment are with the authority of the MHA.

Deprivation of Liberty and the MCA

As we have already discussed, everyone has the right not to be deprived of their liberty except in limited cases specified in the Article (including those of 'unsound mind') and provided there is a proper legal basis in law for the arrest or detention. With no statutory definition of deprivation of liberty (DoL), the first question is, therefore, *what is* a deprivation of liberty? Prior to the Supreme Court judgment[13] in the cases of *Cheshire West* and *P & Q* (involving three people with learning disabilities), there was a marked lack of consistency both in practice and in the courts when deciding whether a person's liberty was 'deprived' or 'restricted'. The judgment has clarified what is to be determined as a deprivation of liberty (we are not suggesting that it's now always easy to decide – uncertainties remain). The important issues are: (a) is the person 'under the complete supervision and control of those caring for her and not free to leave the place where she lives' (the so-called 'acid test'); and (b) is the state responsible? If you are going to compare the situation of the person with that of someone else, the comparison is not with a person with a similar level of disability, but with a healthy person. The purpose of the control, the relative normality of the setting and whether or not the person is compliant are all irrelevant. As Lady Hale put it, 'a gilded cage is still a cage'.[14] This has markedly broadened the scope of a deprivation of liberty and so led to a very considerable increase in the number of people requiring some form of legal scheme to authorise their care.

One remaining question is how long does the person need to be confined in this way before they are deemed to be deprived of their liberty? The Supreme Court did not answer this. It is worth noting that, in one case,[15] a young man with autism was restrained by the police for 40 minutes and this was found to have been a deprivation of liberty. Therefore, considering 'the type, duration, effects and manner of implementation of the measure in question', the more complete the restrictions imposed, the shorter the duration of time before a deprivation ensues.

After the European Court of Human Rights' ruling in Mr L[16] (Chapter 2), the 'Bournewood Gap' was recognised. This referred to the legal predicament of tens of thousands of people who lacked capacity to consent to admission or care and who were deprived of their liberty without the protection of the law. The government (in England and Wales) had to plug this legal gap and introduced the Deprivation of Liberty Safeguards (DoLS) to the MCA. The DoLS scheme is not considered to be fit for purpose[17] and (under the Mental Capacity (Amendment) Act 2019) is to be replaced by the Liberty Protection Safeguards (LPS). The reviewed Code of Practice is still being drafted at the time of writing and therefore the detail of how LPS will operate is not available (and in any event is beyond the scope of this book). When the LPS comes into force, both the DoLS and the LPS will run concurrently for a period, and therefore a brief summary of both schemes is set out below. In the DoLS scheme:

- The person must be aged 18 or over (the age assessment). This is because a person under 18 may be deprived of their liberty using the authority of the Children Act 1989.

- The deprivation of liberty must not have been refused by a health and welfare attorney or a court (the no-refusals assessment).
- The person must lack capacity in relation to the decision about the deprivation of liberty (the mental capacity assessment).
- The person must have a disorder or disability of their mind (the mental health assessment). Note that the definition is the same as for the MHA and *not* the same as for the rest of the MCA.
- The person must not be detained under the MHA at the time or be subject to MHA restrictions that would conflict with the DoLS requirement (the eligibility assessment). It is self-evident that it would be unreasonable, if a person were required to live in a care home under a guardianship order, for example, simultaneously to require them to reside in a care home under a DoLS requirement!
- It must be in the person's best interests to be deprived of their liberty (the best interests assessment).
- The local authority acts as the supervisory body which is responsible for allocating DoLs assessors and giving the standard authorisation.

Registered Medical Practitioners (RMP), if approved as DoLS assessors, may undertake the mental capacity, mental health and eligibility assessments. An Registered Medical Practitioner who wishes to make the eligibility assessment must be both a DoLS assessor and section 12 approved. The Best Interests Assessor (known as the BIA) must be a social worker, nurse (mental health or learning disability), clinical psychologist or occupational therapist, and approved as a DoLS assessor. A BIA may undertake any assessment other than the 'mental health' assessment. A BIA who wishes to carry out the 'eligibility' assessment must also be an Approved Mental Health Professional. See Brindle and Branton[18] for a fuller description of DoLS.

Liberty Protection Safeguards:

- The LPS does not contain any new definition of liberty. It is still being interpreted as set out in Article 5 of the ECHR.
- *Responsible Bodies (RBs)* will replace the supervisory bodies that currently exist in DoLS and will now include NHS Trusts, Clinical Commissioning Groups (CCGs) and Local Authorities.

Responsible Bodies (RBs) in the Liberty Protection Safeguards (LPS)	
Health/care provision	LPS stipulation concerning Responsible Bodies
NHS hospital care	The hospital managers of the NHS Trust will be responsible for authorising any deprivation of liberty that arises in their hospitals
Continuing healthcare funded care	The Responsible Bodies will be the funding CCG
Care homes/hospices	The Local Authority who is meeting the person's needs or in whose area the person is ordinarily resident
Independent hospitals	The Responsible Body is the 'responsible local authority' in England (normally the authority meeting the person's needs or in whose area the hospital is situated)

- LPS will cover those individuals who are aged 16 and 17 in addition to adults, making the legislation consistent with the MCA.
- LPS can be authorised in any environment where the deprivation of liberty is engaged, e.g. care homes, hospitals, sheltered and supported accommodation, and also in a person's private residence.
- A Responsible Body may authorise arrangements if the following authorisation conditions are met:
  - the person lacks the capacity to consent to the arrangements;
  - the person has a mental disorder within the meaning of the MHA; and
  - the arrangements are necessary to prevent harm to the person and proportionate in relation to the likelihood and seriousness of harm to the person.
- The consultation process is essentially the same as the one in DoLS, although the Relevant Person's Representative role has now been replaced by 'an appropriate person'.
- A pre-authorisation review is what provides the process with the required level of independence to be concordant with Article 5. This task can be undertaken by an Approved Mental Capacity Professional (AMCP) or another professional not involved in the person's care. It is expected that the Code of Practice and associated regulations will provide clarity as to who can undertake reviews.
- Where the individual is objecting to care arrangements or is being cared for in an independent hospital, or if the Responsible Body decides to refer the case to an Approved Mental Capacity Profession and and he or she accepts it, the Approved Mental Capacity Professional Responsible Body will need to decide if the individual is objecting or not. Also, the Responsible Body will have to consider the views of the person and any relevant individual about the wishes of the person concerned. Arrangements cannot be authorised unless the pre-authorisation review (and the Approved Mental Capacity Profession) has confirmed that the authorisation conditions are met.

Note

A person can be deprived of their liberty only where:

- it is authorised because the person is detained under the MHA;
- it is authorised by an order of the Court of Protection under section 16(2) of the MCA;
- it is authorised in accordance with the DoLS/LPS procedure set out in Schedule A/AA1 (respectively) of the MCA; or
- it is necessary in order to give life-sustaining treatment, or to carry out a vital act to prevent serious deterioration in a person's condition while a decision with regard to any relevant issue is sought from the court.

Note

DoLS (LPS) must not be used to settle a dispute between a hospital or social services department that wishes to deprive a person of their liberty and a relative who objects. If they cannot be settled amicably, such cases should be decided by the Court of Protection.

The MHA or the MCA

Why, you might ask, have we gone into such detail about the MCA, DoLS and LPS in a book about the MHA? It is because there are now two distinct legislative frameworks (Acts) that can be used to deprive a patient of their liberty in order to provide necessary care and treatment. While the principles, provisions, purposes and policy concerns of the two Acts are quite distinct, both are intended to provide procedural protections for patients. Which you should use is often, but not always, obvious and can be very difficult. In an Upper Tribunal case, Mr Justice Charles highlighted some of the difficulties: 'All decision makers who have to address the application of the provisions of the DoLS contained in Schedules A1 and 1A of the MCA are faced with complicated legislative provisions and their difficulties are compounded when they have to consider the relationship between the MHA and the MCA'.[19]

It is fair to say that Schedule 1A's complexity (persons ineligible to be deprived of their liberty by the MCA) is now infamous. As part of the LPS, Schedule AA1 of the amended MCA will replace Schedules A1 and 1A. Part 7 of Schedule 1AA, 'Excluded arrangements: mental health', takes the place of Schedule 1A. The new terminology does not appear to add further clarity, but the interface, and thereby the decision-making, will be unchanged. The government has indicated that it has no intention to reform the interface at this time.[20]

It doesn't help that judges also appear to change their minds. You may hear the quote from Mr Justice Charles in *GJ* v. *The Foundation Trust and others*,[21] who said: 'The MHA should be considered first, and has primacy. This means the first step should be to see whether or not the patient falls within the scope of the MHA. If they do, the MHA should be used as the means of authorising detention. The MCA should not be considered as an alternative.' He also said that the pivotal issue, in a case where the patient had both a mental and a physical illness, was whether the need for the deprivation was due to the mental or the physical condition. If deprivation of liberty is required because of a mental condition, the MHA should be used; if it is required because of a physical condition, the MCA/DoLS is the correct authorisation. He then acknowledged that both statements are incorrect when he gave judgment in a subsequent case.[22]

For the sake of brevity and clarity, we will limit Justice Charles' statements and provide the following interpretation of the law. We must emphasise that this is our view and we are not lawyers. The difficulty arises from trying to understand the relevant MCA schedule. We have found it helpful to consider what the Department of Health was trying to achieve. Their intention was to try to arrange that the circumstances for using the MHA would be similar for a person who lacks capacity as for a person who retains capacity. If a person retains capacity and consents, then they may be admitted to hospital informally. If they object or resist, then they are deprived of their liberty using the MHA. So, if the person lacks capacity but is compliant, then the MCA/DoLS (the 'lacking capacity' equivalent of informal admission, i.e. not under the MHA) should be used. If the person who lacks capacity objects or resists, then the MHA should be used. This is reflected in the MHA Code of Practice (Chapter 13).

To look at this further, Schedule 1A in brief (and remembering that it is largely incomprehensible to read) says the following.

- If the person is detained under the MHA, then the MCA/DoLS cannot be applied. The person is 'ineligible'.

- If the person is subject to the MHA but is not detained, for example is on a Community Treatment Order (CTO) or guardianship order (or, oddly, on section 17 leave), they can be deprived of their liberty using MCA/DoLS provided that the requirements of the DoLS don't clash with the requirements of the MHA. For example, the patient can't be required to live in care home B under DoLS if they are required to live in care home A under the CTO. The MHA trumps the MCA/DoLS.
- If the person is not subject to the MHA, for example they are living in the community and you've been asked to go and assess them, then they should be admitted under the MCA/DoLS if they are compliant, but under the MHA if they are objecting or resisting.

Notwithstanding, the MHA Code of Practice does offer some guiding principles in relation to which Act to use for both physical and mental disorders and reflects this judgment and further developments in case law. The reader is referred to the English and Welsh Codes of Practice for further details, but the influence of the Supreme Court judgment[23] can be seen, for example, in the following statement (at paragraph 13.53 of the English Code and 13.39 in the Welsh Code) that 'a person who lacks capacity to consent to being accommodated in hospital for care and/or treatment for mental disorder, and who is likely to be deprived of their liberty should never be informally admitted to hospital, whether they are content to be admitted or not'.

So, assuming that use of the DoLS/LPS is not excluded by the prescribed restrictions, it seems to us that there are a number of things to consider:

1. Does the patient need to be in hospital for the assessment or treatment of mental disorder?
2. If the patient has the capacity to make the relevant decisions, do they object to or refuse to consent to either the admission or any part of the required treatment?
3. If the patient lacks the capacity to make the relevant decisions:

   (a) Are they non-compliant with either the admission or any part of the required treatment?
   (b) If they are compliant, would the treatment conflict with that of a valid and applicable advance refusal or refusal by a person with a lasting power of attorney (health and welfare)?
   (c) Is the detention solely for the protection of other people?

If the answer to question 1 and either question 2 or any part of question 3 is yes, the MHA is required.

It is important to note that the Code of Practice discusses 'objection' in the following way: 'Whether a patient is objecting has to be considered in the round, taking into account all the circumstances, so far as they are reasonably ascertainable'. Furthermore: 'In deciding whether a patient objects to being admitted to hospital, or to some or all of the treatment they will receive there for mental disorder, decision-makers should err on the side of caution and, where in doubt, take the position that a patient is objecting.'

If, for treatment of mental disorder in hospital, the patient has capacity and is truly consenting, then informal admission is correct (we say truly consenting because of the number of times patients have said they were persuaded to agree to admission and were told/promised it would only be 'for a day or two'). As an aside, consent requires that patients are told the truth, but also in assessing capacity to consent to admission and treatment one must consider the relevant information needed to make those decisions (one case that considered this was that of a 33-year-old woman, Ms L, with learning disabilities[24]). If the patient lacks capacity but is fully compliant, and there is no valid and applicable advance refusal or conflict with the decision of a person with a lasting power of attorney, then the MCA/DoLS is available.

We acknowledge that this view lacks subtlety and does not take into account all the complexities and nuances of individual cases. We have not included the other issue that the general principles state should be considered, i.e. the least restrictive option. This is because there are arguments on both sides. For example, the rights of appeal are easier and, generally, quicker under the MHA. On the other hand, patients cannot be forced to accept treatment under the MCA/DoLS. The Nearest Relative has rights, including a limited right of discharge, under the MHA, but currently, the patient cannot choose their Nearest Relative, whereas they can choose a person to represent them under the MCA. And so on.

Where there most commonly seems to be a genuine choice between the two schemes, it is not ideal if there is a stand-off between decision-makers under the DoLS (LPS) or the MHA. A common example of this is when discharge is delayed pending implementation of the discharge care plan, relevant decision-making capacity is lacking and a deprivation of liberty requires appropriate authorisation. The MHA Code of Practice guides us in that: 'Decision-makers should also consider whether an individual deprived of their liberty may regain capacity or may have fluctuating capacity. Such a situation is likely to indicate use of the [Mental Health] Act to authorise a deprivation of liberty.' Further to this, the Code says:

> In the relatively small number of cases where detention under the Act and a DoLS authorisation or Court of Protection order are available, this Code of Practice does not seek to preferentially orientate the decision-maker in any given direction. Such a decision should always be made depending on the unique circumstances of each case. Clearly recording the reasons for the final decision made will be important.

That is, show your working! Tribunals will certainly expect you to have considered why the MHA is the preferred legal scheme.

A common query is about whether or not a DoS application is required to transport a patient. The DoLS Code of Practice (we will have to await the updated MCA Code) states:

> Transporting a person who lacks capacity from their home, or another location, to a hospital or care home will not usually amount to a deprivation of liberty (for example, to take them to hospital by ambulance in an emergency). Even where there is an expectation that the person will be deprived of liberty within the care home or hospital, it is unlikely that the journey itself will constitute a deprivation of liberty so that an authorisation is needed before the journey commences.[25]

In a case in which a patient refused to return to a care home, the court[26] confirmed that sections 5 and 6 of the MCA would usually give the necessary authority.

Note

A patient can be deprived of their liberty under the MCA without the use of DoLS, but only if: the deprivation of liberty is wholly or partly for the purpose of giving the person life-sustaining treatment or doing any vital act, and the deprivation of liberty is necessary in order to give the life-sustaining treatment or do the vital act.

The concept of the 'acid test' has evolved in how it was applied differently in a case in 2017.[27] The case involved an in-patient in an Intensive Care Unit who was unconscious and unable to consent to medical care. The Court of Appeal decided that there was no deprivation of liberty because the care was no different from that which anyone without a mental impairment would require: 'The root cause of any loss of liberty was her physical condition, not any restrictions imposed by the hospital.' This means that deprivation of liberty may be interpreted differently depending on the situation.

This judgment has wider implications in mental health settings. For example, in dementia hospital in-patient care, individuals may be both detained under the MHA and receiving end-of-life care. Under such circumstances, it may be necessary to consider:

- whether the restrictions are being imposed owing to the patient's *physical* condition;
- whether the treatment would be materially different from that offered to a patient with capacity in similar circumstances; and
- whether the purpose is for the administration of life-saving treatment.

It may be that the patient's legal predicament has changed and requirement for the use of the MHA should be reviewed. Such decisions should form part of any discussion regarding ongoing care plans and if in doubt practitioners should seek advice from the organisation's legal department.

There are many other routine clinical situations which are encountered that again have not been specifically considered by the courts, but are potential legal traps. Patients with delirium will likely experience impaired capacity regarding treatment and care at some point and the acid test will often be met. It may be that the circumstances are sufficiently differentiated from the situation in *Ferreira* that Article 5 is engaged. The practical outcome is that only people with delirium who are declining treatment or trying to leave tend to be managed under DoLS (or the LPS). Furthermore, objectively the correct legal scheme to authorise the deprivation in many instances will be the MHA, justified because there is a level of risk to others. Again, practically, it is relatively rare for the MHA to be deployed unless the level of risk to others is high. The cumbersome nature of the DoLS scheme and seeming disproportionality of using the MHA to authorise a deprivation of liberty under these circumstances means that many deprivations go unauthorised. As things stand, it is difficult to provide general guidance other than manage each case on its merits, but continue to assess capacity and make decisions on an individual basis. It is noteworthy that damages have been awarded for false imprisonment by a hospital trust when a DoLS authorisation should have been in place.[28] Although there were other complicating factors to this case, it highlights the importance for Hospital Trusts and other health and social care providers to comply with the requirements of the MCA. Whether a more streamlined process under the LPS will resolve this legal predicament remains to be seen.

There are further issues relating to the interface between the MHA and the MCA that need to be mentioned.[29] Patients detained under the MHA may be deprived of their liberty and given treatment for their mental disorder. Physical illnesses unrelated to their mental disorder are treated either with the authority of the patient's capacitous consent or under the MCA. A physically ill patient who lacks capacity and can only be treated if they are deprived of their liberty will be made subject to DoLS. But suppose one has a patient, detained under the MHA, who has a physical illness unrelated to the mental disorder and treatment of which requires deprivation of liberty? The DoLS can't be applied because the patient is detained under the MHA. Can this patient be treated for their physical disorder using the deprivation of liberty authority provided by the MHA (the MCA authorising the actual treatment)? It seems not. The case concerned an Iranian man (a doctor) who lost his application to stay in the United Kingdom and went on hunger strike. He was diagnosed as suffering from either delusional disorder or paranoid personality disorder and detained under the MHA. His Responsible Clinician thought the refusal to eat was unrelated to his mental disorder, saying:

> The purpose of the section 3 admission is so we can administer appropriate psychotropic drugs via the nasogastric tube. We do not see food as treatment for his mental illness. The administration of food via the nasogastric tube has not made a difference to his underlying mental state and indeed his mood has deteriorated. The food is administered to prevent him from dying ... In my view, it is extremely difficult to disentangle how much of his hunger strike is due to underlying depression or possible delusional disorder. It is important to note that, when he was previously treated with antipsychotics and there was a marked improvement in his mental state, there was still no change in his views regarding continuing with the hunger strike. At the moment it is helpful to separate out what we see as treatment for any possible mental health disorder (i.e. psychotropic medication) from medical treatment required to keep him alive.[30]

The judge accepted this:

> On this point I have found the views articulated by the treating clinicians, and in particular Dr WJ, persuasive. She does not consider that the administration of artificial nutrition and hydration to Dr A in the circumstances of this case to be a medical treatment for his mental disorder, but rather for a physical disorder that arises from his decision to refuse food. That decision is, of course, flawed in part because his mental disorder deprives him of the capacity to use and weigh information relevant to the decision. The physical disorder is thus in part a consequence of his mental disorder, but, in my judgement, it is not obviously either a manifestation or a symptom of the mental disorder. This case is thus distinguishable from both the Croydon case and Brady.

He went on:

> ... it will be seen that this might make it impossible for someone to be treated in a way that is outwith his 'treatment' under the MHA if that treatment involves a deprivation of liberty. To take a stark example: if someone detained under section 3 is suffering from gangrene so as to require an amputation in his best interests and objects to that operation, so that it could only be carried [out] by depriving him of his liberty, that process could not prima facie be carried out either under the MHA or under the MCA. This difficulty potentially opens a gap every bit as troublesome as that identified in the Bournewood case itself.

Three alternatives were considered:

- The necessary feeding and associated measures can be taken under the MHA. There is therefore no need for an order under the MCA.
- If the necessary feeding and associated measures cannot be taken under the MHA, an order can and should be made under the MCA interpreted in accordance with the Human Rights Act 1998.
- If the necessary feeding or associated measures cannot be taken under the MHA or the MCA, an order should be made under the High Court's inherent jurisdiction.

The court authorised the deprivation of liberty and treatment under its 'inherent jurisdiction' (see Chapter 1).

A more recent case involved a 34-year-old woman detained under section 3 who required surgery for an aortic aneurysm, but needed to have her teeth removed first. The medical plan involved keeping the patient in hospital for 5 days between the dental and cardiac surgery. Throughout the process she would require restraint and sedation. She lacked capacity to consent to any of the treatment. In other words, the patient would be deprived of her liberty. The court rightly noted that the physical disorder was neither a cause nor consequence of the mental disorder and she could not, therefore, be deprived of her liberty using the authority of the MHA, but wrongly concluded that the DoLS procedure of the MCA was not available.[31] This is because the patient was granted section 17 leave to the general hospital for her surgery. Patients subject to, but not detained in hospital under, the MHA can additionally be placed under DoLS. The DoLS Code of Practice states that: 'People on leave of absence from detention under the Mental Health Act 1983 or subject to supervised community treatment or conditional discharge are, however, eligible for deprivation of liberty safeguards if they require treatment in hospital for a physical disorder.' This was confirmed by Mr Justice Mostyn at a subsequent hearing. It should, however, be noted that:

> If the proposed authorisation relates to deprivation of liberty in a hospital wholly or partly for the purpose of treatment for mental disorder, then the person will also not be eligible if they are: currently on leave of absence from detention under the [1983 Act] or subject to supervised community treatment, or subject to conditional discharge, in which case powers of recall under the Mental Health Act should be used.[32]

Note

A person can be deprived of there liberty only where:

- It is authorised because the person is detained under the MHA;
- It is authorised by an order of the Court of Protection under section 16(2) of the MCA;
- It is authorised in accordance with the DoLS procedure set out in Schedule A1 of the MCA; or
- It is necessary in order to give life sustaining treatment, or to carry out a vital act to prevent serious deterioration in a person's condition while a decision with respect to any relevant issue is sought from the court.

The Mental Health Act

Who's Involved?

First, some titles and common abbreviations.

- **Registered Medical Practitioner (RMP)** We generally use the term Registered Medical Practitioner in this text, in preference to the more common 'doctor', in order to avoid confusion with other professionals who may be entitled to use the latter title. Registered Medical Practitioners carrying out duties under the MHA need a licence to practise from the General Medical Council. The only exception is when they are acting solely as Medical Members of the Mental Health Tribunal, for whom registration alone is sufficient. Depending on the task, the MHA may require any Registered Medical Practitioner or a section-12-approved Registered Medical Practitioner or the Registered Medical Practitioner in charge of the case.

- **Section-12-approved doctor** A Registered Medical Practitioner who is approved, under section 12 of the MHA, by the Secretary of State or another person or organisation under authority given by the Secretary of State as having special experience in the diagnosis or treatment of mental disorder (see Chapter 11).

- **Approved Clinician (AC)** A Registered Medical Practitioner or nurse, psychologist, occupational therapist or social worker of the appropriate class, who has the necessary competencies and has been approved as an Approved Clinician (by the Secretary of State or another person or organisation under authority given by the Secretary of State). Approved Clinicians who are Registered Medical Practitioners are automatically approved under section 12 of the MHA. Approved Clinicians, whether Registered Medical Practitioners or not, are authorised to be 'in charge of the treatment' of an informal in-patient and so may make a recommendation under section 5(2) of the MHA. Only Registered Medical Practitioners may fulfil this role without being Approved Clinicians.

- **Responsible Clinician (RC)** An Approved Clinician who has a detained or Community Treatment Order patient under their care. All hospitals and NHS Trusts that detain patients under the MHA should have a policy that describes how an Approved Clinician is appointed as a Responsible Clinician to a particular patient, both initially and as the patient moves through the service (e.g. becomes a Community Treatment Order patient).

- Many hospital policies use the term Responsible Clinician when they mean the consultant in charge of an in-patient. This is wrong. Only patients subject to compulsion under the MHA have a Responsible Clinician (and not all of them – patients held on a brief order, such as section 5(2), 5(4) or 136, do not have a

Responsible Clinician). Detained and Community Treatment Order patients must have a Responsible Clinician at all times.

- There used to be an assumption that patients were under the care of a single named consultant at all times (the consultant's name would be at the head of the bed in general hospitals) other than, perhaps, when the consultant was on annual leave. Whether or not this continues to be a tenable position with the 40-hour week and times when the consultant or Approved Clinician from another profession is and isn't on call is up to employing organisations. What is clear is that there must be an identifiable, and potentially available, Responsible Clinician out of hours and whenever the patient's usual Responsible Clinician isn't available (some Trust policies, for example, transfer Responsible Clinician responsibilities, out of hours, to the duty consultant psychiatrist). Having said this, a patient can have only one Responsible Clinician at a time. The policies of all detaining authorities should enable easy identification of the Responsible Clinician for all qualifying patients. Only Approved Clinicians can be appointed Responsible Clinicians.

- A detained patient may, in addition to having a Responsible Clinician, have one or more other Approved Clinicians in charge of different aspects of their treatment. Only Approved Clinicians can be in charge of a treatment for a detained patient. This is most likely to occur if a detained patient is prescribed medication for mental disorder and the Responsible Clinician is neither a Registered Medical Practitioner nor a nurse prescriber.

- **Nominated Deputy (ND)** A Registered Medical Practitioner (who need not be an Approved Clinician) or an Approved Clinician (from any of the qualifying professions) who has been nominated by the Registered Medical Practitioner (from any medical specialty) or Approved Clinician in charge of the care of an informal in-patient to act on their behalf in relation to section 5(2). To put it another way: any Registered Medical Practitioner may be a Nominated Deputy, but only a Registered Medical Practitioner in charge of informal patients may nominate a Deputy. Therefore, pre-registration FY1 doctors cannot be nominated deputies. Members of the other professions can fulfil these roles only if they are Approved Clinicians.

- Many hospital policies incorrectly refer to a Nominated Deputy when they mean the consultant's deputy or, even more misleading, the Responsible Clinician's deputy. A Responsible Clinician does not have a Nominated Deputy because a Responsible Clinician is only Responsible Clinician to patients who are already detained (and so a Nominated Deputy would be superfluous). The Nominated Deputy is a position that exists only in relation to section 5.

- A Registered Medical Practitioner/Approved Clinician in charge of informal patients can have only one Nominated Deputy at a time per hospital (if the Practitioner/ Clinician works in two or more hospitals, they can have a Nominated Deputy in each hospital). One Nominated Deputy cannot nominate another. The Nominated Deputy must be 'on the staff' of the same hospital as the nominator.

- **Approved Mental Health Professional (AMHP)** Usually a social worker, but may be a nurse, occupational therapist or psychologist who has received appropriate training and is approved by the local authority. A Registered Medical Practitioner cannot become an Approved Mental Health Professional.

- **Nearest Relative (NR)** This person is determined by a set list in the MHA (section 26). It starts with the patient's spouse or civil partner, then children (if over the age of 18 and whoever is eldest), then parents (the elder one) and so on. The Nearest Relative can be changed by the courts, but only on specified grounds, at the request of the Approved Mental Health Professional or the patient. The responsibility for identifying the patient's Nearest Relative rests with the Approved Mental Health Professional. The Nearest Relative can: be the applicant for sections 2, 3 and 4; stop a section 3 from being applied by objecting to it; and discharge the patient from sections 2 and 3, 37 and Community Treatment Orders (although the Responsible Clinician can override this under certain circumstances).
- **Supervised Community Treatment/Community Treatment Order (SCT/CTO)** The terms have been used interchangeably, although 'CTO' is now the one that is applied. They refer to the MHA power for compulsion in the community. The MHA itself refers only to 'community treatment orders' and 'community patients'. Patients on CTOs are not 'detained' under the MHA. Nor, in European Convention on Human Rights terminology, are they deprived of their liberty.
- **Hospital Manager (HM)** In England, NHS hospitals are managed by NHS Trusts and NHS Foundation Trusts. For these hospitals, the trusts themselves are defined as the Hospital Managers for the purposes of the Act. In an independent hospital, the person(s) in whose name the hospital is registered are the Hospital Managers (in Wales, for a hospital vested in a Local Health Board, it is the Board members). It is the Hospital Managers who are responsible for detaining patients and for the authority of CTOs.
- Hospital managers have a wide range of responsibilities, including: checking the validity of detention and CTO papers, transferring patients between detaining authorities, referring detained/CTO patients to the Tribunal and hearing appeals against detention (and discharging patients from detention). In practice, they delegate most of the responsibilities to MHA administrators and nursing staff and, in relation to hearing appeals, to a group of people specifically appointed for this purpose.
- **Second Opinion Appointed Doctor (SOAD)** A Registered Medical Practitioner, invariably a psychiatrist of some experience, accepted onto a panel by the Care Quality Commission (CQC) and appointed by the CQC to provide a statutory second opinion for medical treatment for a detained patient. The Registered Medical Practitioner becomes an 'actual SOAD' (as opposed to a 'virtual SOAD') only when appointed by the CQC to examine a named detained or CTO patient (see Chapter 8).
- **First-Tier Tribunal of the Health, Education and Social Care chamber** Also called a First-Tier Tribunal (Mental Health) or Mental Health Tribunal or just FTT. Whatever they're called, they are the Tribunals to which detained, CTO and guardianship patients can appeal against their order. For ease, we will call it a Mental Health Tribunal or just a Tribunal.
- **Upper Tribunal** The higher 'appeal court' of the Tribunal service.
- **Medical Member of the Tribunal (MM).**
- **Liable to be detained** This is a confusing term which is often misunderstood. It does not mean patients who meet the criteria for detention but are not subject to the MHA. It refers to patients who are actually detained under the MHA, those on

section 17 leave or absent without leave and those on conditional discharge from a restriction order. It does not include patients on CTOs, despite such patients being subject to recall in a very similar way to those on conditional discharge.

Before looking at different sections of the MHA, it is worth considering the medical role. We think it is helpful to do so from two different angles, historical and current.

The Medical Role in Detention

During the nineteenth century, there was a massive expansion in the population of the United Kingdom's mental hospitals. Patients were taken to the asylums, usually by their relatives, for a variety of reasons, many of which would not be considered acceptable today. Some asylum superintendents (they were not medically trained) accepted such people as patients in part because the size of their salary was determined by the number of residents in their asylum. In 1845, James Luke Hansard (whose father was the first printer to Parliament, hence the official record of Parliament being called 'Hansard') formed the Alleged Lunatics' Friend Society for the 'protection of the British subject from unjust confinement on the grounds of mental derangement'.

The cost of the massive expansion in numbers, and complaints about the grounds for detention, led to demands for restrictions and in 1890 Parliament passed the Lunacy Act. This Act stopped all informal admissions to mental hospitals (other than to Bethlem Royal) and required that two doctors certified that the person was mentally ill enough to warrant admission before the patient could be accepted (except in an emergency). Thus, the medical role was to prevent admission unless the patient was found to be sufficiently mentally disordered to warrant it. The relative would ask for permission to have the patient admitted. The doctors would decide whether the patient met the medical criteria. Only when the relative had two medical 'recommendations' could they approach the hospital superintendent and apply for admission. The relative has (in most cases) been replaced by the Approved Mental Health Professional, but the medical role is largely unchanged to this day. Registered Medical Practitioners (the doctors) often don't see things quite like this, because commonly they already know the patient, but it does help clarify the medical role and explain why the Approved Mental Health Professional cannot make the application for detention until they have two medical recommendations.

The requirement for all patients to be 'certified' was partially removed by the Mental Treatment Act 1930, in that it permitted patients to self-certify (and if you had signed yourself in, you could sign yourself out). The need for 'certification' for voluntary patients was finally removed by the Mental Health Act 1959.

Detaining a patient is often referred to as 'sectioning' them, and we refer to 'sectioned' patients. The term was introduced as it was thought to be less stigmatising than 'certifying'. Detaining and detention are more appropriate words.

Of course, one big difference nowadays from the situation prior to 1959 is that most patients with mental health problems are treated in the community. Furthermore, if they need admission to hospital, for the majority of patients this is consensual and therefore informal (although in some inner-city in-patient wards, the majority of patients are detained under the MHA). As section 131 of the MHA states:

> Nothing in this Act shall be construed as preventing a patient who requires treatment for mental disorder from being admitted to any hospital or registered establishment in pursuance of arrangements made in that behalf and without any application, order or

direction rendering him liable to be detained under this Act, or from remaining in any hospital or registered establishment in pursuance of such arrangements after he has ceased to be so liable to be detained.

That's the MHA's way of saying that patients can be admitted to, and remain in, hospital without use of the MHA!

An alternative way of considering the medical role is as follows. A patient visits a doctor, who examines them and recommends an intervention, be it treatment or admission to hospital. The patient and doctor may discuss options and agree a way forward. If the patient declines to accept the medical advice, and has the capacity to make that decision, then that is, in most circumstances, the end of the matter. But if the patient suffers from a mental disorder and the doctor believes that the risks are sufficient, the doctor can say to an Approved Mental Health Professional, or the patient's Nearest Relative, that the patient has declined help, but nonetheless the doctor thinks it necessary for the patient to be admitted to hospital for the recommended assessment and/or treatment. The Approved Mental Health Professional (or Nearest Relative) may make the decision to agree to admission on behalf of the patient. The patient can then be detained and the treatment given. That is why the MHA is called an 'enabling Act'. It enables clinicians to give treatment to a patient when, without the MHA, the patient's refusal would have to be accepted.

The Structure of the MHA

The Act is divided into chapters called Parts. Part I is very short (one section) and describes the purpose of the Act ('the reception, care and treatment of mentally disordered patients . . . and other related matters'). Part II includes sections relating to civil detention and compulsion, Part III contains court and prison transfer sections, Part IV is about consent to treatment and Part V is about Tribunals. Other parts deal with cross-border arrangements, offences, police powers, advocates, publication of a Code of Practice and many relatively minor matters.

There is also an MHA Code of Practice – two actually, one for England (which was revised in 2015)[1] and one for Wales (which is currently under revision).[2] The Act requires all professionals when performing duties under the Act to have regard to the relevant Code. Importantly, the Codes set out principles that the Secretary of State thinks should inform decisions made under the Act. The principles for England are briefly described below. The MHA Code of Practice gives full details (for the Welsh equivalent, see Appendix 1, section A1.2).

Least restrictive option and maximising independence
Where it is possible to treat a patient safely and lawfully without detaining them under the MHA, the patient should not be detained. Wherever possible, a patient's independence should be encouraged and supported, with a focus on promoting recovery.

Empowerment and involvement
Patients should be fully involved in decisions about their care, support and treatment. The views of families, carers and others, if appropriate, should be fully considered when taking decisions. Where decisions are taken that are contradictory to views expressed, professionals should explain the reasons for this.

Respect and dignity
Patients, their families and carers should be treated with respect and dignity and listened to by professionals.

Purpose and effectiveness
Decisions about care and treatment should be appropriate to the patient, have clear therapeutic aims and promote recovery, and should be performed to current national guidelines and/or current best practice guidelines.

Efficiency and equity
Providers, commissioners and other relevant organisations should work together to ensure that commissioning and provision of mental healthcare services are of high quality and are given equal priority to physical health and social care services. All relevant services should work together to facilitate timely, safe and supportive discharge from detention.

Independent Mental Health Advocates

Patients are entitled to the support of an Independent Mental Health Advocate (IMHA), to help them obtain information, understand and exercise their rights regarding their detention, treatment, appeals and so on, in relation to the MHA if they are:

- detained (other than under sections 4, 5, 135 and 136) (the scope is extended in Wales: see Appendix 1, section A1.1);
- subject to a CTO;
- conditionally discharged;
- subject to a guardianship order;
- informal patients who are being considered for treatment under section 57 or, if under 18 years of age, section 58A.

The range of 'qualifying patients', i.e. those entitled to an Independent Mental Health Advocate, has been extended in Wales (see Appendix 1, section A1.1).

Chapter 5

The Mental Health Act: Part II (Civil Sections)

Section 2 – Admission for Assessment

- Requires two Registered Medical Practitioners – one section 12 approved, the other with previous knowledge of the patient if practicable – and an applicant (Approved Mental Health Professional or Nearest Relative).
- Grounds – see 'Grounds for Detention under Sections 2 and 3' below.

Section 3 – Admission for Treatment

- Requires two Registered Medical Practitioners – one section 12 approved, the other with previous knowledge of the patient if practicable – and an applicant (Approved Mental Health Professional or Nearest Relative).
- The Nearest Relative must not object to the application (positive agreement is not required).
- Grounds – see 'Grounds for Detention under Sections 2 and 3' below.

Section 4 – Admission for Assessment in Cases of Emergency

- Requires one Registered Medical Practitioner and an applicant (Approved Mental Health Professional or Nearest Relative).
- Grounds – Urgent necessity for the patient to be detained under section 2 and waiting to complete section 2 would cause an undesirable delay.

Section 5(2) – Application in Respect of Patient Already in Hospital

- Requires the Registered Medical Practitioner or Approved Clinician in charge of the patient or their Nominated Deputy.
- Grounds – The Responsible Medical Practitioner/Approved Clinician in charge or their Nominated Deputy believes an application under Part 2 (a section 2 or 3) ought to be made.

Section 7 – Application for Guardianship (Aged 16 and over)

- Requires two Registered Medical Practitioners – one section 12 approved, the other with previous knowledge of the patient if practicable – and an applicant (Approved Mental Health Professional or Nearest Relative).
- Grounds – The patient suffers from a mental disorder of a nature or degree that warrants reception into guardianship in the interests of the welfare of the patient or for the protection of other persons.

Grounds for Detention under Sections 2 and 3

In essence, the grounds are similar apart from the 'appropriate treatment' test. The person must suffer from, or appear to suffer from, a mental disorder (or the MHA wouldn't be relevant), that disorder must cause some sort of risk for the person or other people (or there's no need to intervene), the risk can't be assessed or managed without the person being in hospital (we can't detain someone in hospital if they don't need to be in hospital) and the person isn't agreeing to the admission (or they wouldn't need detaining).

Please note, we are referring here to 'detention in hospital' – detention does not include CTOs or guardianship.

Terminology

Mental Disorder

Mental disorder is defined in the MHA as 'any disorder or disability of the mind', a very broad definition indeed. It was decided not to use any of the recognised classification systems because 'diagnoses' in those systems keep changing with subsequent editions. Nonetheless, the International Classification of Diseases (ICD) and the Diagnostic and Statistical Manual of Mental Disorders (DSM) are helpful guides. Affective, schizophrenic and delusional, neurotic, stress-related and somatoform (such as anxiety, phobias, obsessive–compulsive), post-traumatic and hypochondriacal disorders are included. So are organic, personality and eating disorders, mental and behavioural disorders caused by psychoactive substance use, non-organic sleep and sexual disorders, autism-spectrum disorders, and behavioural and emotional disorders in children and adolescents. The MHA Codes of Practice[1] give further guidance.

The definition of mental disorder has two caveats.

- First, dependency on alcohol or drugs is excluded from the definition and so patients cannot be detained if they suffer solely from such dependency. Other conditions relating to alcohol or drug misuse, such as intoxication or withdrawal, are not excluded. Nor are patients excluded if they suffer from such dependency and another mental disorder.

- Second, people with a learning disability and no (other) mental disorder can be detained only if the disability is associated with abnormally aggressive or seriously irresponsible behaviour. (This caveat does not apply for sections 2 and 4.)

Learning Disability

The term 'learning disability' is used throughout the book. We recognise that many clinicians, and others, are more familiar with or prefer the term intellectual disability. We are using learning disability because it is the term used and defined in the MHA ('a state of arrested or incomplete development of the mind which includes significant impairment of intelligence and social functioning') and used throughout the secondary legislation and Codes of Practice.

Nature or Degree

To explain the difference, we can do no better than quote the judge in R. v. Mental Health Review Tribunal for the South Thames Region, ex p. Smith:[2]

Although the wording of this phrase is disjunctive ['or' not 'and'] the nature and degree of the patient's mental disorder will be inevitably bound up so that it matters not whether the issue is dealt with under nature or degree. The word 'nature' refers to the particular mental disorder from which the patient suffers, its chronicity, its prognosis and the patient's previous response to receiving treatment for the disorder [the judge rejected the view that 'nature' is static] and the word 'degree' refers to the current manifestation of the patient's disorder.

It is not unusual for Tribunal judges to ask the Responsible Clinician whether it is the nature or degree of the patient's mental disorder that leads to the requirement for detention. The answer is usually both, if only because they are 'inevitably bound up'.

Health or Safety or Protection of Other Persons

This should be self-explanatory, but seems to be misunderstood. It is quite different from the often-expressed grounds for detaining someone under the MHA, i.e. dangerousness. It is perfectly proper and lawful to detain a patient solely because 'it is necessary for his health'.

In Hospital

This bit is more important than may be first apparent. A patient cannot be detained under the MHA unless they need to be in hospital. That is why, when completing the documentation, we have to say why other interventions (e.g. in the community) won't be adequate to achieve the necessary assessment or treatment. As discussed earlier (Chapter 1, 'Interpretation of the MHA'), this is relevant in relation to section 17 leave of absence and renewal of the detention order. It is also relevant when thinking about recall of a CTO patient.

It is surprising how often there are arguments over what a hospital is. Section 145 of the MHA defines 'hospital' to include 'any health service hospital within the meaning of the National Health Service Act 2006', which in turn includes 'any institution for the reception and treatment of persons suffering from illness' and any 'clinics, dispensaries and out-patient departments maintained in connection with any such . . . institution'.

Medical Treatment

This term is much broader than would be expected from general usage. It includes 'nursing, psychological intervention and specialist mental health habilitation [learning new skills], rehabilitation [relearning lost skills] and care'. The word 'specialist' mustn't be ignored. For example, in a case in which a patient with Korsakoff's psychosis had to be stopped from drinking alcohol, it 'would require tactics of general distraction and diversion to prevent Mr N obtaining alcohol. Even if that would amount to care, it is not care within the definition of treatment, because it would not be "specialist mental health . . . care."'[3] Furthermore, the MHA allows the detention of a person for the receipt of appropriate treatment only if 'the purpose of [the treatment] is to alleviate, or prevent a worsening of, the disorder or one or more of its symptoms or manifestations'.

Does there have to be a clear evidence base for this 'purpose' test to be met or can it rest on the personal view of the doctor making the section 3 recommendation? Suppose the patient has failed to respond to the treatment in the past, can one still maintain that the purpose of the intervention is to alleviate or prevent a worsening? If the patient's condition continues to deteriorate despite treatment, does this mean that the 'purpose' test should fail? These are questions we have been asked.

Although it is true that exactly what is meant by 'purpose' isn't clear, it seems to us that such questions should be answered in the same way as clinicians have always decided whether or not to recommend a medical intervention for a patient. These are clinical decisions.

Appropriate Medical Treatment Is Available

This criterion only applies to treatment orders, e.g. sections 3 and 37. This term is explained in the MHA as follows: 'references to appropriate medical treatment, in relation to a person suffering from mental disorder, are references to medical treatment which is appropriate in his case, taking into account the nature and degree of the mental disorder and all other circumstances of his case'.

The MHA Codes of Practice clarify this in a number of ways.

- Any medical treatment provided must always be an appropriate response to the patient's condition and situation and, wherever possible, should be the most appropriate treatment available. It may be that a single medical treatment does not address every aspect of a patient's mental disorder.
- Medical treatment that aims merely to prevent a disorder worsening is unlikely, in general, to be appropriate in cases where normal treatment approaches would aim (and be expected) to alleviate the patient's condition significantly. However, for some patients with persistent and severe mental disorders, management of the undesirable effects of their disorder may be the most that can realistically be hoped for.
- Appropriate medical treatment does not have to involve medication or psychological therapy – although it very often will. For some patients, appropriate treatment might consist only of nursing and specialist day-to-day care under the clinical supervision of an Approved Clinician in a safe and secure therapeutic environment with a structured regime.

We assume what counts as appropriate (medical) treatment in differing circumstances and for different conditions will continue to be challenged in, and clarified by, the courts. At the time of writing, there have been a number of cases that have all said the same thing. It is agreed that appropriate treatment is more than just locking a person up, but in none of the cases was it decided that appropriate treatment wasn't being provided. The threshold is low and we haven't yet had a case in which the court decided that appropriate treatment was not being provided.

The cases where the 'appropriate treatment' test is challenged tend to be when the patient is detained on the grounds of a personality disorder and is refusing all interventions. The Upper Tribunal pointed out that the definition of medical treatment in section 145 'is sufficiently broad to include attempts by nursing staff to encourage the patient to engage by taking what the NICE Guidance calls "a positive and rewarding approach [which] is more likely to be successful than a punitive approach in engaging and retaining people in treatment". This is not difficult to satisfy'.[4] The judge said that the Tribunal should explore the issues with the following questions:

> 39. *What precisely is the treatment that can be provided?* This requires the tribunal to make a finding on the particular treatment that is available rather than resorting to general

statements. It ensures that the tribunal makes particularised and individualised findings in respect of the particular patient. That is what the legislation requires; it is consistent with the Code.

40. *What discernible benefit may it have on this patient?* This complements the previous question. Although section 145 defines treatment widely, there is a common thread that runs through all the elements: its purpose must be to confer some benefit on the patient, if only to the extent of preventing the patient's condition getting worse. And the answer must relate to the individual patient, not to patients generally. This does not reintroduce the treatability test. It merely restates what section 145 says. It concentrates on what can be attained, not on what will or may be attained.

41. *Is that benefit related to the patient's mental disorder or to some unrelated problem?* This question is concerned with the relationship between the treatment and the patient's disorder. The treatment must be available for the disorder. It is not permissible to detain a patient who has both a personality disorder and diabetes in order to treat the latter but not the former. That is what the statute provides. This would not be appropriate medical treatment for section 72(1)(b)(iia); nor would it be appropriate to detain a patient in these circumstances for section 72(1)(b)(i).

42. *Is the patient truly resistant to engagement?* This addresses the patient's argument directly. The tribunal may find, despite assertions to the contrary, that the patient is prepared to engage. Or it may find, again despite assertions to the contrary, that the patient may yet be brought to engage. In either case, this finding will remove one element of the patient's argument, although it is still necessary to decide whether there is some form of treatment that would be available and appropriate. If the tribunal finds that the patient is not prepared to engage and will never be brought to engage, that will not necessarily be decisive. This is because the definition of treatment is so broad that it includes much that does not require the patient's engagement in formal therapy.

43. I do not say that the tribunal must set out the answers to those questions in every case. That will depend on the issues raised before the tribunal and on the evidence. Nor do I say that those are the only questions that may be relevant. . . . What other questions arise will again depend on the issues raised and the evidence. They might include: What would be the purpose of the proposed treatment? Is it actually available? Will it produce a significantly better outcome than the present position? Does it have adverse effects that outweigh its benefits?

In one Upper Tribunal hearing the judge made it clear as to what evidence the Tribunal would accept. The Responsible Clinician argued there was no appropriate treatment available for a patient, also diagnosed with a personality disorder. A variety of treatments had been tried but nothing had worked, it was also argued that the ward environment was unsuitable and the Responsible Clinician's preferred option was that the patient be transferred to another hospital. The patient submitted that the tribunal was obliged to accept that evidence and should be discharged. He was however, prescribed medication for mental disorder and his mental state was being managed, to a degree, by nursing staff. The judge rejected the arguments and, amongst other things, decided that 'it will be a matter for the judgment of the tribunal if the point has been reached where the medical treatment given to a patient is no longer appropriate'.[5]

But, as we said previously, the threshold is low and there hasn't yet been a case in which the court decided that appropriate treatment wasn't being provided. A specific question, raised in a 2013 case,[6] was: 'Is the nature of the risk posed by a patient detained under the MHA relevant to the appropriateness of the treatment under section?' The patient (as with all cases challenging whether appropriate treatment is available) was diagnosed with 'dissocial or antisocial personality disorder'.

> The court looked at the criteria:
>
> (b) the tribunal shall direct the discharge of a patient liable to be detained otherwise than under section 2 above if it is not satisfied—
>
> > (i) that he is then suffering from mental disorder or from mental disorder of a nature or degree which makes it appropriate for him to be liable to be detained in a hospital for medical treatment; or
> >
> > (ii) that it is necessary for the health of [sic] safety of the patient or for the protection of other persons that he should receive such treatment; or
> >
> > (iia) that appropriate medical treatment is available for him; ...[7]
>
> and noted that risk was clearly relevant to (i) and (ii). The judge went on to say that risk may also be relevant to appropriate treatment, giving the analogy 'a patient with a life-threatening condition may be prescribed treatment that would not be appropriate for a patient with a less serious condition'.

Use of the Mental Health Act in a General Hospital

The MHA makes no distinction between 'mental health/psychiatric' and 'general' hospitals. They are all just hospitals. In practice, however, there may be several major differences.

Most general hospitals do not employ Approved Clinicians and cannot therefore appoint a Responsible Clinician. If general hospitals are to detain patients, i.e. be the detaining authority, there must be some arrangement, such as a service-level agreement, to enable Approved Clinicians from a local mental health hospital to be appointed as Responsible Clinicians within the general hospital. Patients cannot be transferred to a general hospital under section 19 (Regulations as to transfer of patients) unless a Responsible Clinician can be appointed. This does not stop transfer under section 17, i.e. on leave of absence.

The general hospital also needs to identify MHA 'Hospital Managers', who have the training and skills required to hear appeals against detention, and administrators, again with the necessary training and support. We are aware of arrangements whereby the services of mental health trust personnel are used for these purposes.

More difficult is where general hospitals aren't registered with the Care Quality Commission to take detained patients. It is important to note that it is unlawful to use section 5(2) in these hospitals because there are no Hospital Managers to whom the section 5(2) report can be 'furnished'.

The Process

It doesn't matter who starts the process (general practitioner, psychiatrist, nurse, social worker, relative, etc.). The patient, for sections 2 and 3 (the most common), must be examined by two Registered Medical Practitioners, who make and date medical recommendations, on or before the date the Approved Mental Health Professional makes an application. The Codes of Practice require the Registered Medical Practitioners to make a 'direct personal examination of the patient and their mental state'.

If neither Registered Medical Practitioner has previous knowledge of the patient – previous attendance at, for example, a case conference about the patient would count as 'previous knowledge' – then it is recommended that both Registered Medical Practitioners should be section 12 approved. There must be no more than 5 days between the two medical examinations. The days on which the medical examinations are made aren't counted. So if the first medical recommendation is made on a Monday, the second must be made on or before the following Sunday. If the two Registered Medical Practitioners examine the patient at the same time, they may, if they wish, make a joint recommendation on the appropriate form. Otherwise they must each make separate recommendations. The Approved Mental Health Professional then has 14 days from the second medical examination in which to personally see and make an application (for section 4, the application must be made within 24 hours).

Section 12(1) provides that the medical recommendations required 'shall be given by practitioners who have personally examined the patient'. Furthermore, the MHA Code of Practice states that a medical examination for these purposes must involve 'direct personal examination of the patient and their mental state'. A judgment published during the Covid-19 pandemic overturned the guidance permitting online video MHA assessments by doctors and Approved Mental Health Practitioners.[8]

Both Codes of Practice state that it is the doctor's responsibility to find a bed. This will be on behalf of the hospital. Most hospitals have 'bed-managers' of one sort or another. This also means you have to think about the type of bed (acute, psychiatric intensive care, medium secure, etc.) required. All other responsibilities lie with the Approved Mental Health Professional. These include identifying and consulting the Nearest Relative (although if a Registered Medical Practitioner knows the Nearest Relative then preliminary discussion would be helpful), transporting the patient to hospital, making sure children and pets are properly cared for (we're aware of one case when a farmer was detained and the Approved Mental Health Professional had to make arrangements for 300 cows – installing a tenant farmer resolved the problem) and ensuring that the patient's home is secure. The Codes recommend using the ambulance service to take the patient to hospital, with police support, if necessary, to ensure safety.

Although there is no legal obligation for either Registered Medical Practitioner to stay with the Approved Mental Health Professional, it is important for good relationships and may be necessary initially for safety. At the very least, discussion with the Approved Mental Health Professional before leaving is essential.

When going to a patient's home to undertake an MHA assessment, safety is paramount. Never go alone. It is helpful to have a 'pack' you take with you: maps or 'sat-nav', a copy of the Code of Practice (and/or this book!), a notebook, paper and detention papers, a mobile phone and important telephone numbers. In this day and age, a smartphone would be sufficient for many of these functions. It's essential to make sure you know who is likely to be in the house, who is going to go with you or meet you there and, if the latter, where you're going to park and meet. Are the police required? Always take your ID and be honest and open about your role. You have no right to enter private premises without permission. If the patient asks you to leave before your assessment is completed, you should do so. Lord Parker said: 'Unless it is to be said that a householder is to sit down and submit, not only to his liberty being infringed in his own house, but also to assault by injection, and to his liberty being removed in hospital, I cannot say that to hit out with a fist is an unreasonable use of force.'[9] You would not be trespassing if a co-owner gave you permission to stay.

Note

Specialist skills or facilities may be needed to undertake assessment of particular patients. Children, those who don't have English as a first language, patients with a severe learning disability or deafness, or those who present particular risks are examples. You should not undertake assessments for which you do not have the necessary training or experience. This does not mean that you should walk away – you should, of course, help identify an appropriate person or service and assist with the urgent needs of the patient in the meantime. But it is OK (and good practice) to say that you are not qualified to make an assessment.

Section 2 or Section 3?

The MHA Codes of Practice give guidance on whether section 2 or section 3 is most appropriate. The amended Code for England has changed the emphasis so as to encourage less use of section 2 and more of section 3.

Section 2 should only be used if:

- the full extent of the nature and degree of a patient's condition is unclear;
- there is a need to carry out an initial in-patient assessment in order to formulate a treatment plan or to reach a judgment about whether the patient will accept treatment on a voluntary basis following admission; or
- there is a need to carry out a new in-patient assessment in order to reformulate a treatment plan or to reach a judgment about whether the patient will accept treatment on a voluntary basis.

Section 3 should be used if:

- the patient is already detained under section 2 (detention under section 2 cannot be renewed by a new section 2 application); or
- the nature and current degree of the patient's mental disorder, the essential elements of the treatment plan to be followed and the likelihood of the patient accepting treatment as an informal patient are already sufficiently established to make it unnecessary to undertake a new assessment under section 2.

The Code for Wales is given in Appendix 1, section A1.3.

But there is another matter to consider: the patient's Nearest Relative can prevent application of a section 3 by objecting to it. On the one hand, it is considered improper to use a section 2 rather than section 3 simply because the Nearest Relative might object. The Code of Practice (England) states that:

> Consultation must not be avoided purely because it is thought that the nearest relative might object to the application ... If the nearest relative objects to an application being made for admission for treatment under section 3, the application cannot be made. If it is thought necessary to proceed with the application to ensure the patient's safety and the nearest relative cannot be persuaded to agree, the AMHP will need to consider applying to the county court for the nearest relative's displacement under section 29 of the Act.

The Welsh Code is stronger (see Appendix 1, section A1.4).

On the other hand, if the application is for section 2, the detention can go ahead, despite the Nearest Relative's objection. The patient is then safe and treatment can start while a decision is made as to whether or not there are grounds to request displacement of the Nearest Relative and a court hearing is organised. If the application is for section 3, however, the patient would remain in the community while the application to court for displacement was made. We would be interested in the views of the courts, should a patient, or others, come to serious harm that was predicted by the clinicians and could have been avoided by the use of section 2. This is one of many unanswered legal questions.

As is discussed in Chapter 8 on consent to treatment, there is no difference between section 2 and section 3 in terms of what treatment can be given to the patient.

Additional Points

- The usual team of two Registered Medical Practitioners and an Approved Mental Health Professional must not usually (see below) have defined conflicts of interest for personal (e.g. they are first-degree relatives), professional (e.g. in the same team or one directs the other) or business reasons (e.g. business partners). The full list for England and Wales is in their Codes of Practice and in Appendix 1, section A1.5 for Wales and Appendix 2, section A2.1 for England. Although the information is given in the Codes of Practice, it is taken from Statutory Instruments[10, 11] and is therefore law rather than guidance. However, the Code of Practice has added, under 'financial conflict': 'It is also good practice for doctors on the staff of an NHS trust or NHS foundation trust to ensure that one of the recommendations is given by a doctor not on the staff of that trust'. Given the common requirement for both doctors to be section 12 approved, because the patient is not known to either doctor, and given the geographical scope of many NHS Trusts, we have doubts as to the ability of the NHS to comply with this. Oddly, but usefully, the MHA Reference Guide[12] states that: 'The final word "trust" in the last sentence of the paragraph should be read as hospital i.e. a single site hospital, rather than a multi-site trust.'
- If the choice is between a section 4, avoiding all conflicts of interest, or a section 2 or 3 but all three assessors work in the same team, then a section 2 or 3 is the preferred option (England only).
- If the application is for detention in an independent (fee-paying) hospital, then only one of the Registered Medical Practitioners may be employed by that hospital (in England – in Wales neither may be employed by the independent hospital).
- Although an Approved Mental Health Professional is the preferred applicant, an application can be made by the patient's Nearest Relative.
- Patients can be moved, using the authority of the MHA, between hospitals only if they are detained by reason of an application. Section 4 patients, like sections 2 and 3, have an applicant. Patients held under section 5(2) do not have an applicant.
- Section 5(4) is known as the nurse's holding power. A nurse 'of the prescribed class' (a qualified mental health or learning disability nurse) can detain for up to 6 hours a patient who is 'receiving treatment for mental disorder as an in-patient'. This is to hold the patient until a section 5(2) can be applied.
- In section 5(2), what is an in-patient? The Code of Practice defines it as 'a person who is receiving in-patient treatment in a hospital'. This excludes out-patients and those receiving treatment in accident and emergency departments. In one case, the judge said that the word 'suggests the allocation and use of a hospital bed'.[13]

- Patients held under section 5 can be restrained, but not treated, using the authority of Part IV of the MHA. Medical treatment is either with the patient's consent, if they retain decision-making capacity, or under the MCA if they lack capacity in relation to that decision and the MCA criteria are met.
- The authority to transport the patient to hospital under section 2, 3 or 4 comes from the application, founded on the medical recommendation(s).
- Hospitals are not required to accept patients. The patient is formally detained in hospital only when the papers are accepted by the Hospital Managers (in practice, this is usually a nurse on the ward, the MHA administrator or medical records staff, on behalf of the Hospital Managers).
- Detaining a patient takes time. Can the patient be held while the process is being completed? As noted below, there was a case in which a woman was held in a section 136 suite for 13 hours, under the authority of the MCA until, following assessments, she was detained under section 2 of the MHA. Using the MCA for this purpose was deemed to be illegal. The judge said that Part II of the MHA *provides a comprehensive code for compulsory admission to hospital for non-compliant incapacitous patients such as the claimant. The common law principle of necessity does not apply in this context.* However, in addition to pointing out that section 4 should be used if the circumstances are urgent, the court reassuringly went on to say: 'each case necessarily turns on its own facts. However in our view it is unlikely in the ordinary case that there will be a false imprisonment at common law or deprivation of liberty for the purposes of Article 5(1) ECHR if there is no undue delay during the processing of an application under ss.2 or 4 MHA for admission'.[14]

When Do the Sections End and Who Can End Them?

- **Section 2** after 28 days, or earlier if discharged by the Responsible Clinician, Nearest Relative, Hospital Managers or Tribunal.
- **Section 3** after 6 months, or later if the section has been renewed or the patient is absent without leave, or earlier if discharged by the Responsible Clinician, Nearest Relative, Hospital Managers or Tribunal.
- **Section 4** after 72 hours, or earlier if discharged by the Responsible Clinician, or later if the section 4 has already been converted to a section 2 by the addition of the relevant additional medical recommendation (it may or may not require a section-12-approved Registered Medical Practitioner, depending on who made the section 4 medical recommendation). If converted to a section 2, then the date of commencement of the section 2 is backdated, i.e. it is deemed to have started when the section 4 started.
- **Section 5(4)** after 6 hours, or earlier if a Registered Medical Practitioner or Approved Clinician who can furnish a report under section 5(4) arrives 'at the place where the patient is detained' (this is rather odd, as it means the time at which the Registered Medical Practitioner/Approved Clinician arrives on the ward rather than when they have made a decision whether or not to complete a section 5(2)).
- **Section 5(2)** after 72 hours, or earlier if the patient is detained under section 2 or 3, or as soon as any one of the team who assess the patient decides not to proceed with a section 2 or 3, or if the patient is moved from the hospital where they are held. The

Code of Practice states that section 5(2) 'should not be used to continue to detain patients after the doctor or Approved Clinician decides that, in fact, no assessment for a possible application needs to be carried out or a decision is taken not to make an application for the patient's detention'.

Additional Points

- The Nearest Relative must give 72 hours' notice of their intention to discharge the patient from detention or from a Community Treatment Order, in writing, to the Hospital Managers. The 72 hours starts when the letter is received by an authorised person on behalf of the Hospital Managers, or, if posted, when the letter is received by the hospital or when placed in the internal post. Given the 72-hour limitation on giving the Responsible Clinician time to consider whether or not to issue a barring order (see next point below), it is essential that hospitals have a procedure in place should the Nearest Relative leave the written request with staff on the ward.

- The Nearest Relative's power to discharge the patient can be overridden by the Responsible Clinician issuing what is called a barring order. The Responsible Clinician can do this only if they believe that the patient, if discharged, 'would be likely to act in a manner dangerous to other persons or himself'. This is a different threshold from the 'for the health or safety of the patient or for the protection of other persons' criterion. The barring order lasts for 6 months, whether or not the patient goes on to another section or becomes informal and is then re-detained.

- If the Responsible Clinician issues a barring order in relation to a Nearest Relative request for discharge of a patient on section 3, then the Nearest Relative may apply for a Tribunal review.

- A Nearest Relative request for discharge from guardianship cannot be barred, nor is there a requirement to give 72 hours' notice (a Nearest Relative cannot discharge Part III guardianship patients).

- A court can 'displace' the Nearest Relative, and authorise another person as the patient's Nearest Relative, if the Nearest Relative 'unreasonably objects' to a section 3 or guardianship order or 'has exercised without due regard to the welfare of the patient or the interests of the public' their power to discharge the patient (section 29 of the MHA).

Sections 135 and 136

Although sections 135 and 136 aren't in Part II of the MHA, we include them in this chapter because they are commonly met in general psychiatric practice.

Section 135 – Warrant to Search for and Remove Patients

- Subsection (1) permits an Approved Mental Health Professional to obtain a warrant authorising a police officer to enter premises where:

  there is reasonable cause to suspect that a person believed to be suffering from mental disorder –

  (a) has been, or is being, ill-treated, neglected or kept otherwise than under proper control, in any place within the jurisdiction of the justice, or

  (b) being unable to care for himself, is living alone in any such place.

- Subsection (2) enables a warrant authorising a police officer to enter premises to 'take or retake' a patient who is already detained under the MHA.

Notes

- Under section 135(1), a section 135 cannot be executed on the grounds of the person being 'unable to care for himself' unless the individual is living alone.
- The phrase 'or kept otherwise than under proper control' is offensive and should have been amended.

Section 136 – Mentally Disordered Persons Found in Public Places

This section enables a police officer to remove to a 'place of safety' someone they find 'in a place to which the public have access ... who appears to be suffering from mental disorder and to be in immediate need of care or control'. In October 2017, the Department of Health and the Home Office published guidance to support the implementation of changes to the police powers and places of safety provisions in the MHA[15] (made by the Policing and Crime Act 2017). The main changes implemented are summarised as follows:

- section 136 powers may now be exercised anywhere other than in a private dwelling;
- it is now unlawful to use a police station as a place of safety for anyone under the age of 18 in any circumstances;
- a police station can now only be used as a place of safety for adults in specific circumstances, which are set out in regulations;
- the maximum detention period is 24 hours (unless a doctor certifies that an extension of up to a further 12 hours is necessary);
- before exercising a section 136 power police officers must, where practicable, consult one of the health professionals listed in section 136(1C), or in regulations made under that provision;
- a person subject to section 135 or 136 can be kept at, as well as removed to, a place of safety.
- a new search power allows police officers to search persons subject to section 135 or 136 powers for protective purposes.

Sections 135 and 136

The purpose of both sections is to take patients to a place of safety. What is considered a place of safety has now been broadened to include: a hospital; an independent hospital or care home for mentally disordered persons; a police station; residential accommodation provided by a local social services authority; any other suitable place (with the consent of a person managing or residing at that place). The preferred place of safety, unless the patient is too violent or physically ill, is usually a dedicated place (often called a 136 suite) within a mental health service. Both police stations and accident and emergency departments may be used as places of safety (but only if the patient is too disturbed or in need of medical treatment respectively).

Both sections last up to 24 hours, to enable the patient to be assessed for their mental health needs, including the need for detention under section 2 or 3. The patient may be moved from one place of safety to another within the 24 hours.

The detention ends when the patient is detained under section 2 or 3 or as soon as one of the team (a Registered Medical Practitioner or Approved Mental Health Professional) who assesses the patient decides not to proceed with a section 2 or 3. However, if the patient has not yet seen an Approved Mental Health Professional, they should be offered the opportunity to see one. The patient may be offered, and accept, informal admission to hospital, or community mental health or social care help.

The key points of this chapter thus far are summarised in Table 5.1.

Note

With regard to a non-compliant incapacitous patient: in a recent case, the police entered a woman's house and took her to a section 136 suite using the authority of the Mental Capacity Act. She was held there for 13 hours until, following assessments, she was detained under section 2 of the Mental Health Act. Using the MCA to do that for which the MHA is intended was deemed to be illegal. The MCA cannot be used by the police to remove people to hospital or other places of safety for the purposes set out in sections 135 and 136 of the MHA. Further, the judge said that Part II of the MHA provides a comprehensive code for compulsory admission to hospital for non-compliant incapacitous patients such as the claimant. The common law principle of necessity does not apply in this context.

Filling in the Forms

Medical recommendation forms are very well designed. The instructions are simple and the required information is clear. It is surprising, therefore, how many errors are made.

- Make sure you put your name in the box for the doctor and the patient's name in the box for the patient. It is not unusual for the names to be in the wrong boxes.
- If the patient's name is unknown, this should be stated and a brief description of the patient given, e.g. 'White male aged approximately 35'. The American custom of making up a name for unidentified people (bodies), usually John or Jane Doe, is not accepted practice in England and Wales. If a name is made up, it must be clear that this is an alias. The patient's name and address must be the same on all forms.
- The forms require your full name. So if you have a very embarrassing middle name that you wish to keep secret, don't put in your initial and no one will ask!
- Where there are choices, such as 'in the interests of the patient's own health', or 'in the interests of the patient's own safety' or 'with a view to the protection of other persons', the form asks that options that do not apply should be deleted. Do not tick the options you want to keep.
- Clinical information, the evidence that indicates that the patient suffers from a mental disorder, should be jargon free where possible and emphasise symptoms, signs and behaviours. 'Known schizophrenic' is not helpful (nor is it polite).
- There is a requirement to explain why the patient needs to be in hospital, i.e. why the patient cannot be managed safely in the community and why informal admission is not possible
- If the recommendation is for section 3 detention, there is a requirement to list the hospital(s), or units within the hospital(s), at which the appropriate treatment is

Table 5.1 Key information governing the detention of patients under Part II or sections 135 or 136 of the Mental Health Act

	Section 2	Section 3	Section 4	Section 5(2)	Section 135	Section 136
By whom?	Section-12-approved RMP plus another RMP plus an AMHP or NR. One RMP should have previous knowledge of the patient if practicable	Section-12-approved RMP plus another RMP plus an AMHP or NR. One RMP should have previous knowledge of the patient if practicable	RMP plus AMHP or NR	AC or RMP in charge of the patient, or their ND	Magistrate plus AMHP (and police constable and RMP)	Police constable
Where?	Patient anywhere (but should not be on a CTO)	Patient anywhere (but should not be on a CTO)	Patient anywhere (but should not be on a CTO)	Patient an in-patient in hospital (*not* in an A&E department) and not on a CTO	Person in premises specified in the warrant	Person anywhere other than in a private dwelling and its associated buildings or grounds
For how long?	28 days	6 months	72 hours	72 hours	24 hours	24 hours
First criterion	Mental disorder	Mental disorder	Urgent necessity for the patient to be detained under section 2	RMP/AC/ND believes that an application under Part II (section 2 or 3) should be made	Mental disorder	Mental disorder
Second criterion	Disorder of a nature or degree that warrants the detention of the patient in hospital	Disorder of a nature or degree that makes it appropriate for the patient to receive medical treatment in hospital	Waiting to complete section 2 would cause an undesirable delay		The person is ill-treated, neglected, 'kept other than under proper control' or unable to care for themselves	Person is in immediate need of care or control

55

Table 5.1 (cont.)

	Section 2	Section 3	Section 4	Section 5(2)	Section 135	Section 136
First purpose	Hospital detention for assessment (followed by treatment)	Hospital detention for medical treatment			To gain access to private premises and to provide a place of safety	To provide a place of safety and to permit assessment
Second purpose (and also a criterion)	In the interests of the patient's health or safety or for the protection of other persons	It is necessary for the patient's health or safety or for the protection of other persons			To permit assessment	In the interests of the person or for the protection of other persons
Final criterion		Appropriate treatment is available				
Medical treatment with MHA authority	Yes	Yes	No	No	No	No
Appeal	To Tribunal within first 14 days and/or to HMs	To Tribunal any time, and/or to HMs	No right of appeal	No right of appeal	No right of appeal	No right of appeal
Renew	Not renewable	Renewable	Not renewable	Not renewable	Not renewable	Renewable
CTO	Cannot progress to a CTO	Can progress to a CTO	Cannot progress to a CTO	Cannot progress to a CTO	Cannot progress to a CTO	Cannot progress to a CTO

A&E, accident and emergency; AC, Approved Clinician; AMHP, Approved Mental Health Practitioner; CTO, Community Treatment Order; HM, Hospital Manager; ND, Nominated Deputy; NR, Nearest Relative; RMP, Registered Medical Practitioner.

available. The patient can be detained only to one of the hospitals/units listed. If the whereabouts of an available bed is not known, then either the list must include the eventual location of the bed or the form cannot be completed until the bed is found.

- Although a joint medical recommendation may be completed if both Registered Medical Practitioners examine the patient at the same time, bear in mind that errors in the clinical information cannot be corrected on joint recommendations.
- Hospitals may, if they wish, copy or design and print their own forms. However, the wording on the form must be that which is in the legislation.
- An amendment to regulations[16] enables many of the statutory forms under the MHA to be communicated electronically (England only). Guidance on this is now available from the Department of Health and Social Care.[17] Notably, at the time of writing, not all trusts have technical infrastructure in place to deal with electronic submissions of section papers.

The relevant forms for England and Wales are listed in Appendices A2.2 and A1.14 respectively.

Section 15 – Rectification of Applications and Recommendations

All detention papers should be scrutinised by the mental health legislation or medical records department, on behalf of the Hospital Managers. In many hospitals, the medical recommendations are also scrutinised by Registered Medical Practitioners. The purpose of this is to correct rectifiable errors (not all errors are rectifiable) quickly so that the patient is, and remains, lawfully detained. Corrections, including submitting a new medical recommendation (unless a joint medical recommendation form was used), can be made, with the permission of the Hospital Managers (always given), within 14 days of the application. It is essential, therefore, that the relevant department can quickly contact all Registered Medical Practitioners who make medical recommendations so that forms may be amended within the permitted timescale.

Section 17 – Leave of Absence from Hospital

The Responsible Clinician can send a detained patient on leave from the hospital. This does not apply to patients on many Part III (forensic) sections, e.g. section 35, 36 or restriction orders. Also, patients held on sections 5(2), 5(4), 135 and 136 do not have a Responsible Clinician and so cannot be sent on leave. Section 17 leave is not required for the patient to leave the ward, provided that they remain in the hospital (this isn't to suggest that there shouldn't be proper assessments and a clear authority for a patient to be given time away from the ward). Section 17 leave can be granted only by the patient's Responsible Clinician. The duty cannot be delegated. There is no Nominated Deputy. It can't be delegated to nursing staff: 'Leave at nurses' discretion' written in the notes is unlawful. Leave can be authorised in advance for a specified date, for a single specified period, for repeated days or purposes. Conditions as to where the patient can, or can't, go can be applied. The leave may be granted for the patient to go out alone, or only with the attendance of hospital staff or with other conditions. It can be authorised with a statement that the leave can be withdrawn at the nurses' discretion, but such withdrawal is allowed only before the leave starts. If the proposed period of leave exceeds 7 days, then the Responsible Clinician must consider a CTO.

A common question is whether or not senior psychiatric trainees can grant section 17 leave. The answer is, almost always, no. Only Responsible Clinicians can grant leave, and to be appointed as Responsible Clinician for a patient the doctor has to be an Approved Clinician. Although a senior trainee could become an Approved Clinician, it is very unlikely they would do so (unless they are already on the General Medical Council's Specialist Register for psychiatry or are in their final trainee year and are in a locum consultant post – see Chapter 11).

Only the Responsible Clinician can recall a patient from section 17 leave. The recall must be in writing. If the patient doesn't return, they are deemed to be absent without leave (AWOL).

Additional Points

- Section 17 leave can be used to enable a detained patient to attend a general hospital for treatment of a physical disorder. However, a patient cannot be admitted 'nominally' to a mental health unit and sent immediately on section 17 leave. This is because a patient cannot be detained under section 2, 3 or 4 unless they need to be in hospital for assessment and/or treatment of their mental disorder. The patient cannot need this if they can be immediately sent on leave. Transfer to a general hospital, under section 19, for treatment of both the mental and physical disorders would be perfectly proper, as would initially detaining the patient to the general hospital (i.e. the general hospital is named on the application and, for section 3, named on the medical recommendations), again for assessment or treatment of both disorders. If the patient is to be detained to the general hospital on section 2, 3 or 4 (or via section 19 transfer), the general hospital, as the detaining authority, will need to appoint a Responsible Clinician. Many general hospitals will not have Approved Clinicians on their staff and will need to have an arrangement with their local mental health hospital.
- It is essential if considering transferring a patient to a general hospital for treatment of a physical illness, whether the patient is detained or not, to consider the authority being used for ensuring that the patient's rights are respected with regard to consent to treatment. The rules are discussed in detail in Chapters 3 and 8. For the moment, it is important to consider whether the patient is being treated:
  - with the authority of the MHA (for mental disorder); or
  - with the authority of the MCA, in their best interests because they lack capacity in relation to that decision and there is no substitute authority under the MCA; or
  - with the patient's consent as a capacitous individual; or
  - with the authority of the parent or guardian of an under-16-year-old who lacks competence.
- Where a single site has hospital buildings managed by different NHS Trusts, section 17 leave is required if the patient is to leave the building to which they are detained and enter the other Trust's grounds or another building.
- Patients detained under a number of Part III MHA orders (patients involved in criminal proceedings or under sentence) – see Chapter 6 – cannot be granted section 17 leave by the Responsible Clinician. Depending on the section, they may need to

return to court to request leave or need the additional permission of the Ministry of Justice.

- Although section 17 applies only to detained patients, since the decision in the *Rabone* case,[18] very careful consideration must be given to the risk of suicide (and risks to other people) before permitting informal psychiatric patients to leave hospital. The patient took her own life while on leave, having been given permission to go home for the weekend. Of course, given that she was informal, had she been refused permission, it might have been necessary to detain her under the MHA.

Section 18 – Return and Readmission of Patients Absent without Leave

If a detained patient goes AWOL, they remain liable to detention and may be brought back to the hospital until:

- if subject to section 2 – the end of section;
- if subject to section 3 – the end of section or 6 months, whichever is later. If the patient is AWOL for more than 28 days, then, on return, they must be examined within 7 days by the Responsible Clinician to ensure that they continue to meet the criteria for detention. The appropriate statutory form must be completed.

Notes

- The patient may be returned to the hospital by: an Approved Mental Health Professional, any member of the hospital staff, a police officer or anyone authorised in writing by the Hospital Managers.
- If a condition of the leave was that the patient was required to stay in another hospital, then that hospital's staff have the same authority.
- Although others may have the authority to return the patient, and may be called on for assistance, the responsibility for the return lies with the detaining hospital.
- A section 135 warrant is still required to enter private premises to reach a patient who is AWOL. However, there is no requirement for medical evidence to obtain the warrant.

Services designated as low, medium or high security are required to notify the Care Quality Commission, using the relevant form, of any unauthorised absence of a person detained or liable to be detained under the MHA, and of the return of persons from unauthorised absences. It should also be noted that the Commission must also be notified of the death of any patient who dies while detained, or liable to be detained, under the MHA.

Section 19 – Regulations as to Transfer of Patients

Section 19 refers to transfer from one set of Hospital Managers (or local Social Services departments for patients under guardianship) to another. It moves the patient's detention (or CTO) to a different detaining (for CTO patients, 'responsible') authority. It applies only to patients who are 'liable to be detained in a hospital by virtue of an application'. This means that patients held on sections 5(4) or 5(2) can't be transferred under section 19 because they have no applicant (note that patients on section 4 do have an applicant). Section 19 is not required when a patient moves between hospitals managed within one Trust or detaining authority. It is perhaps surprising, but the patient's Responsible Clinician isn't involved in the legal process. Nonetheless, such a move would normally have been arranged as part of the patient's care plan, with which the Responsible Clinician should definitely be involved!

For restricted patients, the permission of the Secretary of State at the Ministry of Justice is required.

If an NHS patient is detained in an independent hospital, the NHS body that has contracted for the patient's care in that hospital can authorise the patient's transfer without the agreement of the managers of the independent hospital.

> **Note**
> Section 19 can also be used to transfer a patient from detention to guardianship.

Section 20 – Duration of Authority

Renewal is another duty placed on the Responsible Clinician that cannot be delegated. If detention is to be renewed, the Responsible Clinician has two months, prior to the end of the section, in which to examine the patient and complete the statutory renewal form, which is then submitted to the Hospital Managers. Before writing the report, the Responsible Clinician must consult with at least one other person who has been professionally concerned with the patient's medical treatment. Following this, another person who is professionally concerned with the patient's treatment and is not of the same profession as the Responsible Clinician must confirm, on the form, agreement with the Responsible Clinician about the need for renewal of the detention and that the patient meets the criteria. The other professional does not need to be an Approved Clinician. It is important to remember that detention can be renewed only if the patient needs to be in, or at, hospital as part of their care plan, in order to receive appropriate medical treatment (unless it is renewal of a CTO).

If the patient is being treated with medication for mental disorder on the authority of a Second Opinion Appointed Doctor certificate (see Chapter 8) or has had electroconvulsive therapy authorised by such a doctor within the period of detention and the patient's detention is to be renewed, then the Responsible Clinician must complete a form provided by, and to be sent to, the Care Quality Commission (section 61 – Review of treatment) at the same time as they complete the renewal form.

The medical report providing 'objective medical expertise' (as required by Article 5 of the European Convention on Human Rights) for the purposes of the renewal of a section is provided by the Responsible Clinician, regardless of their profession. During the 2006 Mental Health Bill's passage through Parliament, before its approved provisions were incorporated into the MHA, there was considerable argument as to whether or not a person who is not medically qualified (i.e. is not a Registered Medical Practitioner) can provide the required 'objective medical expertise'. The Minister argued that the competencies required to become an Approved Clinician mean that Approved Clinicians from any profession will be able to provide the expertise and so meet the European

Convention's requirements. Parliament's Joint Committee on Human Rights (a committee whose role is to advise when it believes Parliament is in danger of passing law that is not compatible with the European Convention) wrote that, in its view, only a Registered Medical Practitioner, and clinical psychologists in certain cases, could provide objective medical expertise.[19, 20] At the time of writing, there has yet to be the inevitable court case to decide the matter.

Section 7 – Application for Guardianship

Guardianship is not used extensively and its use varies considerably from one Social Services authority to another. It may be appropriate when compulsion is needed, but primarily for the patient's welfare rather than their health. The local Social Services authority takes the place of the Hospital Managers.

As with sections 2 and 3, guardianship requires medical recommendations from two Registered Medical Practitioners, one of whom must be section 12 approved. The criterion is that: 'He [the patient] must be suffering from a mental disorder of a nature or degree which warrants his reception into guardianship and it is necessary in the interests of the welfare of the patient or for the protection of other persons.'

The guardian will be appointed or approved by the local Social Services authority. Guardians can:

- decide where the patient must live (this decision overrides the decision of an MCA attorney or court deputy);
- require the patient to attend for medical treatment (but there is no authority to require the patient to accept the treatment), work, training or education;
- require access to the patient to be given to a Registered Medical Practitioner, Approved Mental Health Professional or other relevant person.

The local Social Services will also appoint an Approved Clinician to act as Responsible Clinician for the purpose of renewing or confirming the guardianship order.

As with a section 3 order, the Nearest Relative has a power of veto and would then need to be displaced for a guardianship order to be made. The initial order lasts 6 months, after which it can be renewed for a further 6 months, and then for a year at a time. The patient can appeal to a Mental Health Tribunal once in each period. A guardianship patient may be admitted to hospital informally. If the patient is detained under section 2 or 4, the guardianship continues. Detention under section 3 cancels the guardianship. Patients detained on a section 3 may be transferred to guardianship (section 19) with the relevant application.

Section 19 also authorises guardianship to be transferred to a different guardian (mirroring detention).

Guardianship does not authorise deprivation of liberty. In one case,[21] a person appealed against a guardianship order because it was being used to deprive them of their liberty. The Upper Tribunal pointed out that it was the care plan that deprived the person of their liberty, not the guardianship order. It used to be argued that guardianship was of little use because it did not give the authority to convey the patient to wherever they were required to be. This has been rectified and guardianship now includes the power to convey. Nonetheless, given the provisions of section 5 of the MCA, the authority of a health and welfare attorney or court deputy, the DoLS provisions of the

MCA and CTOs, it is not surprising the number of new guardianship orders has declined from 470 in 206/7 to 55 in 2020/21. The MHA Code of Practice notes that guardianship may be preferable to a CTO where:

- the focus is on the patient's general welfare, rather than specifically on medical treatment;
- there is little risk of the patient needing to be admitted compulsorily and quickly to hospital;
- there is a need for an enforceable power to require the patient to reside at a particular place.

Note

The guardian has an 'exclusive right to decide where a patient should live'. This right cannot be overridden, even by the Court of Protection.

Section 117 – Aftercare

All patients who have been detained under section 3, 37, 45, 47 or 48 are entitled to statutory aftercare. The local Clinical Commissioning Group (CCG) and, where appropriate, the NHS Commissioning Board (in England) or the Local Health Board (in Wales), and the local Social Services authority have a duty to make provision for aftercare services until they (the CCG and the local Social Services authority) are satisfied that the patient no longer needs services. A patient who is settled and well in a care home may still meet the criteria for section 117 aftercare if removal of the provision would, for example, risk readmission to hospital. The Care Act 2014 has clarified that aftercare services are within the remit of section 117 only if they (a) meet a need arising from or related to the person's mental disorder and (b) reduce the risk of a deterioration of the person's mental condition (and so reduce the risk of the person requiring admission to a hospital again for treatment of mental disorder).

This is a statutory right of patients who have been detained under these five sections. Although addressing the section 117 needs of the patient will usually be undertaken within care planning meetings, it is important to record that the patient is subject to section 117. Services provided under section 117 must be provided free of charge to the patient. The responsible local Social Services authority is generally the one in which the patient was resident prior to detention under the MHA. The duty remains until a positive decision is made to end it.

Section 134 – Correspondence of Patients

One issue that we have not addressed in previous editions is that of the correspondence of detained patients. Section 134 outlines when and how a detained patient's post may be withheld. Briefly, the provisions are as follows:

'Postal packets' (mail) from patients may be withheld from posting if:

- someone requests that they do not receive mail from the detained patient;
- the patient is detained in a high-secure hospital and it is thought likely that the contents will cause distress to the recipient or any other person (apart from staff of the hospital) or cause danger to any person.

The Act includes a list of people to whom patients have an absolute right to write, including the Hospital Managers, ministers, the Care Quality Commission, people providing advocacy services, etc. A full list is in the MHA. Postal packets to patients may be inspected and withheld if the patient is in a high-secure hospital and it is thought necessary in the interests of the patient's safety or for protection of other persons.

Mental Health Units (Use of Force) Act 2018

Finally, in this section, nicknamed 'Seni's law', the Mental Health Units (Use of Force) Act is the culmination of campaigning following the death of Seni Lewis, who died (aged 23) after having been restrained on a mental health unit. While it does not amend the MHA, the explicit purpose of this Act is to increase the oversight and management of the use of force in mental health units by imposing a number of requirements around the use of force in such units. In response, there are practical steps that can be implemented by organisations, but the reader is referred to the Act itself for the provisions.[22] The government has conducted a consultation on the statutory guidance supporting the Act;[23] however, regulations are awaited which will determine when the legislation comes into force.

6

Chapter

The Mental Health Act: Part III (Sections Relating to Courts and Prisons)

Unless you use these sections regularly, it is almost impossible to remember the numbers. It's easier to think about the stages in criminal proceedings when transfer to hospital might be required.

The Important Principles

- A court cannot commit a person to hospital under the MHA if the alleged offence is not punishable by imprisonment, i.e. if the person (if guilty) can't be locked up in prison for the offence, then the court can't have them locked up in hospital for it.
- If the person needs medical treatment in hospital for mental disorder, then they should get it. The disorder doesn't need to be connected to the crime; indeed, it may have started long after the offence was committed.

The Situations

A person may:

- need to be sent to hospital following arrest and charge but before they can be tried for an alleged offence:
  - for assessment of a mental disorder – section 35; or
  - for assessment and treatment – section 36;
- have been remanded in prison awaiting trial and need hospital assessment and treatment for mental disorder – section 48 (invariably with a restriction order – section 49: see later);
- have been tried and found guilty, but it is unclear whether or not they should be sentenced to hospital or prison – section 38;
- have been tried, found guilty and the court has decided that the correct 'sentence' (the word used is 'disposal', not a very pleasant term) is to send the person to hospital – section 37 (with or without a restriction order – section 41: see later);
- have been tried, found guilty and the court has decided that the correct sentence is to send the person to prison; while serving the prison sentence, it is decided that the person needs treatment in hospital – section 47 (almost always with a restriction order – section 49: see later).

If a court decides to send the person to hospital, but thinks that there is a serious risk to the public if the patient were to be moved to a less secure hospital or ward than that specified by the court or were to be discharged from hospital altogether, the court will add a restriction order. This prevents the Responsible Clinician from moving, sending on leave or discharging the patient without the permission of the Secretary of State for the Ministry of Justice. This has the section number 41, so you will see patients held on a 37/41.

The Ministry of Justice may add the same restriction to patients transferred from prison (whether on remand or sentenced). This has the section number 49, so you will see patients held on a 47/49 or 48/49.

The Accused

A person may be:

- unfit to plead (i.e. too mentally ill to understand the difference between a plea of guilty and not guilty, or to instruct counsel, or challenge jurors or follow the evidence);
- so seriously mentally ill that they can't be found guilty of the crime of which they are accused because they were unable to form the intent to commit the crime (to be found guilty of most offences, except driving offences, the person must have intended to commit the crime in addition to actually committing it: this is called the *mens rea*); these patients may be sent to hospital under the Criminal Procedure (Insanity and Unfitness to Plead) Act 1991;
- subject to something known as a 'hybrid order', under which the person, having been found guilty, is sent to hospital, but once their mental health has improved, may then be sent to prison to complete their sentence.

Additional Points

- It is lawful, under some circumstances, for a patient to be detained on a forensic section (under Part III) and a civil section (under Part II) at the same time. So, for example, if a patient is admitted from the court for assessment on a section 35 and requires treatment for mental disorder to which they are not consenting, they may be detained on a concurrent section 2.
- A patient detained on a section 37, without a restriction order, can be discharged by the Responsible Clinician at any time, in the same way as a patient on a section 3.
- It is almost unheard of for a patient to be transferred from prison under section 47 or 48 without the section 49 restriction. This is because to do so would put discharge in the hands of the Responsible Clinician rather than the court (for remanded prisoners) or the Ministry of Justice (for sentenced prisoners).
- If a patient transferred from prison with a restriction order is discharged from their section by the Tribunal, they will be transferred back to prison (to await trial if they were on a section 48 or to complete their sentence if on a section 47).
- All sentenced prisoners, except 'lifers', have a date on which they would be discharged from prison. Once this date has passed, a patient detained on a section 47 with a 49 restriction can, and almost always does, continue to be detained. However, the restriction to their discharge (and leave and transfer) by the Responsible Clinician is removed. The patient is said to be detained on a 'notional 37'. That is, the same rules apply as if the patient had been placed by a court on a section 37 without a restriction order.

- Victims have rights to information in relation to certain Part III (forensic) patients who have committed sexual or violent crimes. Patients on a section 37 with a 41 restriction may be granted conditional discharge. This is a sort of halfway house between detention and informality. It has many similarities to a CTO. The patient will have a medical and a social supervisor and may have conditions attached to the conditional discharge.

- Patients on conditional discharge may be admitted to hospital informally, i.e. they remain on conditional discharge. Alternatively, they may be recalled to hospital by the Secretary of State (Ministry of Justice), in which case they again become restricted patients. This is usually because the patient's medical supervisor has said it is necessary (because for some reason the risks are increasing, usually owing to a deterioration in the patient's mental health). The Secretary of State will require a medical report before, or very soon after, the recall.

- An informative but tragic case which illustrates how the different options may apply for people who have been convicted of crimes is that of Mr B.[1] He was diagnosed with autistic spectrum disorder and personality disorder and attempted to kill a young boy by throwing him over the railings of a high platform of the Tate Modern art gallery. Two experts recommended a mental health disposal (disposal is the term used, acknowledging that many are uncomfortable with the terminology), with admission to Broadmoor Hospital under section 37 with a section 41 restriction order as they felt that the therapeutic measures available in hospital would be beneficial. A third expert recommended a criminal justice disposal, i.e. prison, pointing out that he could be transferred to hospital under section 47 (with restrictions under section 49) if the treatment in prison was unsuccessful: 'in other words, whilst the prison system can provide therapeutic provision it also has the flexibility of returning you to maximum security conditions in hospital if necessary.' There was, in fact, a third option, section 45, in which the person is sent first to hospital, then prison once they have recovered sufficiently. In the event, he was sentenced to life imprisonment, i.e. the second option.

A summary of the key points covered in this chapter appears in Table 6.1.

Discharge of Restricted Patients on Conditions that Amount to Deprivation of Liberty

There are some patients on restriction orders who, it is thought, could leave hospital and be safely managed in the community so long as they were subject to such conditions as amount to deprivation of liberty. Unfortunately, there are significant legal problems in granting a conditional discharge to restricted patients with such conditions. The problems started with the Court of Appeal decision in *SSJ* v. *RB*.[2] The court decided there was no provision in the MHA to deprive the man of his liberty once an order for his conditional discharge had been made. The next relevant case was Mr M. The brief details of the case are as follows. Mr M was subject to a hospital order with a restriction (sections 37/41). He applied for a tribunal to request discharge and had capacity to consent to a discharge care package that met the 'acid test' for deprivation of liberty. Ultimately, the Supreme Court held that the MHA does not allow the Tribunal or Secretary of State to order the conditional discharge of a restricted patient to be subject to conditions which amount to a deprivation of liberty.[3]

Table 6.1 Summary of key information governing the detention of patients under Part III of the Mental Health Act

	Section 35	Section 36	Sections 37/41	Section 38	Sections 47/49	Sections 48/49
By whom?	One RMP	Two RMPs (one section-12-approved)	Two RMPs (one section-12-approved)	Two RMPs (one section-12-approved)	Two RMPs (one section-12-approved)	Two RMPs (one section-12-approved)
Can the RC move the patient?	RC cannot move, send on leave or discharge	RC cannot move, send on leave or discharge	RC cannot move, send on leave or discharge (if the patient is restricted)	RC cannot move, send on leave or discharge	RC cannot move, send on leave or discharge	RC cannot move, send on leave or discharge
Can medical treatment be given using the authority of the MHA Part IV?	Cannot give medical treatment for mental disorder without the patient's consent	Can give medication under Part IV	Can give medication under Part IV	Can give medication under Part IV	Can give medication under Part IV	Can give medication under Part IV
How long does the section last?	28 days, up to 12 weeks	28 days, up to 12 weeks	Until discharged by Secretary of State/Tribunal/RC	12 weeks, renewable up to 12 months	Until the end of sentence. Patient remains detained but without restriction	Depends on the outcome of the legal case
Where next for the patient?	Return to court	Return to court	Can be conditionally or absolutely discharged or placed on a CTO	Return to court	Return to prison	Return to prison

CTO, Community Treatment Order; RC, Responsible Clinician; RMP, Registered Medical Practitioner.
Note: Patients detained under Part III treatment orders have the same entitlement to aftercare under section 117 as Part-II-detained patients (see Chapter 4).

Following this, the Secretary of State set out guidance.[4] This is guidance, not law, but it sets out the Secretary of State's proposed solution to the problem posed by the judgment. Regrettably, from the outset, it is worth noting that the position is far from straightforward.

The Secretary of State's guidance distinguishes between patients with and without capacity. Where the patient has capacity to consent to the relevant discharge arrangements that amount to a deprivation of liberty, the placement cannot be authorised either under provisions of the MCA or through the valid consent of the patient. If a patient no longer requires treatment in hospital, but requires constant supervision, the Secretary of State can consider providing his consent to a long-term escorted leave of absence, under section 17(3) of the MHA.

Under section 17(3), a Responsible Clinician (or the Secretary of State for restricted patients) can direct that the patient remains 'in custody' of any person during the leave of absence provided there is written authorisation by the Hospital Managers. This provision means that during the period of leave those who are caring in the hospital or care home may escort the detained person at all times (or impose other safety measures); they may restrain the patient if he or she tries to abscond and the person can be recaptured if he or she escapes.

Since then, the court has considered the case of Mr B.[5] Mr B had been convicted of sexual offences and was subject to a sections 37/41 restriction order. He was conditionally discharged by the Tribunal, 17 years after his conviction. Mr B had the capacity to consent to his care, support and accommodation arrangements and was supervised at all times, including when he was visiting his family. The judge determined that the court's inherent jurisdiction could authorise conditions amounting to a deprivation of a patient's liberty in circumstances where that patient consents to a conditional discharge under the MHA.

In respect of patients lacking capacity, the guidance then breaks that category down into two parts. First, there are those patients whose best interests require a care home or placement and a care plan to help them perform daily living activities or self-care and where the support would amount to a deprivation of liberty. Second, there are those who lack capacity and whose care plan requires a deprivation of liberty primarily to protect the public.

For the first category, the guidance suggests that if the care plan requires deprivation of liberty, the Tribunal can issue a deferred conditional discharge and the necessary arrangements made to put in place Deprivation of Liberty Safeguards (DoLS) or Liberty Protection Safeguards before the patient is discharged.

For the second category, the guidance suggests that a conditional discharge would not be appropriate and section 17(3) leave would be open to consideration with no need for an additional authorisation under the MCA. Despite this, there have been cases whereby judges have decided that deprivation of liberty under the MCA may still be appropriate.

In one case, ZZ, the purpose of the restrictions on the person's liberty was to address, prevent and control his sexual urges.[6] Justice Moor concluded it was lawful, despite the clear risk of causing harm, to deprive him of his liberty using the provisions of the MCA:

> I make it clear to Mr ZZ that I have no doubt that the restrictions upon him are in his best interests. They are designed to keep him out of mischief, to keep him safe and healthy, to keep others safe, to prevent the sort of situation where the relative of a child wanted to do

him serious harm, which I have no doubt was very frightening for him, and they are there to prevent him from getting into serious trouble with the police.

Two further individuals, Mr R and Mr A, were considered together in court of protection proceedings.[7] At the time of the hearing, Mr R was detained under section 37 of the MHA with a section 41 restriction order and conditional discharge was being sought. Mr A had been conditionally discharged after having been convicted of sexual assault. Both patients lacked capacity regarding the relevant aspects of their care and residency and the judge decided that both of them were not 'ineligible' to be deprived of their liberty by the DoLS (with reference to Schedule 1A). In the case of Mr R, the judge said, 'it might be argued that the purpose of the deprivation of liberty and some of the other elements of the care package is the protection of the public, rather than the care of Mr R'. She went on to say:

> In those circumstances the provisions of the care plan in terms of supervision and ultimately deprivation of liberty is, as Moor J put it, 'to keep him out of mischief' and thereby assist in keeping him out of psychiatric hospital. This is strongly in his best interests, as well as being important for reasons of public protection.

The judge then appeared to take issue with the Secretary of State's guidance:

> ... I am not convinced that the division the Secretary of State makes in the Guidance between patients whose care plan is in the patients' best interests, and those where the deprivation of liberty is primarily for the purposes of managing risk to the public, is one that stands up to close scrutiny.

Finally, in relation to the guidance, for patients already on conditional discharge, the following options will be considered: (a) variation of conditions; (b) recall, with or without instantaneous grant of escorted leave to the current placement; (c) absolute discharge; (d) referral to tribunal.

By way of conclusion, for those who have capacity, the inherent jurisdiction is one potential mechanism to effect the conditional discharge of restricted patients into the community under circumstances that amount to deprivation of liberty. However, in the guidance, 'the Secretary of State does not consider that this is the correct approach', and it also runs the risk of being overturned by a higher court in due course. The predicament of those with capacity is therefore currently unclear.

The use of extended section 17 leave for those with or without capacity is not without issues. A recent judgment calls the guidance and practice of authorising long-term community care under section 17(3) into question, particularly when care does not involve a significant part of hospital treatment.[8] Furthermore, many local authorities do not contribute financially to section 117 aftercare while a patient is on section 17 leave, but would do so upon conditional discharge. Local arrangements may require review to take account of this. Hospital Managers will need to ensure that their legal requirements under section 17(3) are met and that there are policies about how to manage these 'virtual patients'.

For the incapacitated restricted patients, there are possible solutions when conditionally discharged with issues around deprivation of liberty utilising the authority of the MCA. Notwithstanding, there will be cases that will rigorously test the boundaries of individual best interests versus public protection.

Community Treatment Orders

Community Treatment Orders (CTOs) continue to be the subject of much debate, partly over the ethics and effectiveness of the provision, neither of which is the subject of this book, and partly over their complexity, which we do need to address. The essence of a CTO is that the Responsible Clinician needs the authority to recall the patient to hospital. The patient will have clinical needs and problems similar to those of a patient who requires detention for medical treatment in hospital, except that they can be managed safely in the community so long as the Responsible Clinician has the power to recall them to hospital. Given the judgments in relation to section 17 leave, outlined in Chapter 1, it could be argued that these needs can be met by the use of section 17 leave. Whether or not this is true, the MHA requires that a CTO must be considered if leave longer than 7 days is to be granted.

> **Note**
>
> The term Supervised Community Treatment, which was used in the previous Code of Practice, but not in the MHA, is not used in the revised Code.

Recommending a CTO

A CTO can be applied only from a non-restricted treatment order. This generally, although not exclusively, means section 3 or 37 of the MHA. Thus:

- the patient must suffer from a mental disorder of a nature or degree that makes it appropriate for them to receive medical treatment;
- it is necessary for their health or safety or for the protection of other persons that they receive such treatment;
- subject to their being liable to be recalled as mentioned below, such treatment can be provided without their continuing to be detained in a hospital;
- it is necessary that the Responsible Clinician should be able to exercise the power to recall the patient to hospital;
- appropriate medical treatment is available for the patient.

The Act states that in deciding whether or not the Responsible Clinician needs the power to recall the patient, the Responsible Clinician

> shall, in particular, consider, having regard to the patient's history of mental disorder and any other relevant factors, what risk there would be of a deterioration of the patient's condition if he were not detained in a hospital (as a result, for example, of his refusing or neglecting to receive the medical treatment he requires for his mental disorder).

So how should one decide whether or not to place a patient on a CTO? If we may give two quotes from Lord Warner (on behalf of the government) during the debate on the Mental Health Bill in the House of Lords in 2007:[1]

> One thing that has not changed as much as we would like, however, is the continuing number of revolving door patients. They leave hospital, disengage from mental health services, do not continue with their treatment, their health deteriorates and they end up compulsorily detained in hospital. We may have differences in view about the numbers involved, but that is the cycle we are trying to deal with.

> On safety, my clear recollection is that distinguished forensic psychiatrist Professor Tony Maden's 2006 review of homicides by patients with severe mental illness concluded that there is a need for legal powers allowing compulsory treatment in the community for patients with a serious mental illness and a history of non-compliance with treatment.

These two quotes help demonstrate a tension in the use of the CTO provision. The first includes: disengagement from services, stopping treatment, deteriorating health and re-detention in hospital. The second adds 'serious mental illness' and a 'history of non-compliance with treatment'.

The Act's criteria for a CTO have none of these requirements spelled out. Balancing patient autonomy (as required by the right to private and family life in Article 8 of the European Convention on Human Rights) with safety and health isn't easy. The Code of Practice for England[2] advises that the Responsible Clinician

> must assess what risk there would be of the patient's condition deteriorating after discharge, for example as a result of refusing or neglecting to receive treatment. A tendency to fail to follow a treatment plan or to discontinue medication in the community, and then relapsing may suggest a risk justifying use of a CTO rather than discharge into community care. Other relevant factors will vary, but are likely to include the patient's current mental state, the patient's capacity to make decisions about their care and treatment and attitude to treatment and risk of relapse, the circumstances into which the patient would be discharged, and the willingness and ability of family and/or carers to provide support (especially where aspects of the care plan depend on them).

The Code advises that 'CTOs should only be used when there is reasonable evidence to suggest there will be benefits to the individual', and gives the following suggestions:

- evidence of a clear link between non-concordance with medication and relapse sufficient to have a significant impact on well-being requiring treatment in hospital;
- clear evidence that there is a positive response to medication without an undue burden of side-effects;
- evidence that the CTO will promote recovery;
- evidence that recall may be necessary (rather than informal admission or reassessment under the Act).

The Welsh Code gives similar guidance – see Appendix 1, section A1.6. The decision is made by the Responsible Clinician and Approved Mental Health Professional.

It is important to understand that a CTO cannot exist independently. The patient's current section, usually a section 3 or 37, continues running underneath. This is why, if a

CTO is revoked, the patient is back on their pre-CTO section. There have now been several occasions when Tribunals have given section 3 patients a deferred discharge, for a few weeks' time, to give the Responsible Clinician time to put the patient on a CTO. Under these circumstances, the CTO is very short-lived because it ends when the section ends. *MP* v. *Mersey Care NHS Trust* illustrates this issue.[3] The patient had been given a deferred discharge by the Tribunal, i.e. that he be discharged 6 weeks after the hearing (to give time for a care plan to be organised). The Tribunal suggested that the Responsible Clinician consider a CTO. But a CTO remains in force only until 'the patient is discharged in pursuance of an order under section 23 . . . or a direction under section 72' (section 17C of the MHA). In other words, the CTO ended at the time the patient's section 3 ended, i.e. at the end of the 6-week period!

> **Note**
>
> When completing the paperwork, the final part of the form must not be signed and dated until the patient is able to leave hospital. Once on a CTO, the patient cannot be detained unless formally recalled from the CTO.

Many services in England and Wales have different teams responsible for in-patients and for patients in the community. This means that the Responsible Clinician, and the team, may change as soon as the patient is placed on a CTO. To avoid patients 'falling through the net', missing legal requirements in relation to consent to treatment or having conditions attached with which the receiving Responsible Clinician and team disagree, liaison between the teams is extremely important. All services should have policies addressing the issue. This is vital when patients are transferred from an in-patient service many miles from the community service (e.g. because the patient had been placed in an out-of-area hospital).

Conditions Placed on a CTO Patient (Section 17B)

All patients on a CTO have two mandatory requirements made of them:

1. that, if they are to be required to take medication for mental disorder, they make themselves available for examination by the Responsible Clinician or Second Opinion Appointed Doctor (as appropriate) to enable a Part 4A certificate to be completed;
2. that they make themselves available for examination by the Responsible Clinician for the purpose of renewing the CTO.

In addition, the Responsible Clinician and Approved Mental Health Professional together may place additional conditions on the patient. These might be to do with where the patient lives, what activities the patient may or may not undertake, requirements in relation to supervision and medication, and anything else they think appropriate, provided that the conditions *do not* amount to deprivation of liberty (see below) and that the conditions are necessary or appropriate for one or more of the following:

- ensuring that the patient receives medical treatment;
- preventing risk of harm to the patient's health or safety;
- protecting other persons.

The conditions should be kept to the minimum necessary to achieve their purpose and they should be clearly expressed so that the patient can understand them. It is essential that the conditions are agreed with the patient. If they aren't, the CTO is almost certain to fail and will therefore be pointless.

Although the conditions can be changed by the Responsible Clinician without reference to an Approved Mental Health Professional, good practice dictates that changes would generally be discussed during Care Programme Approach meetings. It is essential that the patient, and others affected by the changes, are informed (subject to confidentiality rules).

The question of whether a patient's Responsible Clinician could impose conditions in a CTO which amount to a deprivation of liberty was considered by the Supreme Court in the case of Mr J.[4] The Supreme Court unanimously overturned the Court of Appeal judgment, relating to the same man, deciding that the conditions attached to a CTO must not amount to deprivation of liberty. They also considered what the options for the Tribunal are if they determined that a community patient is being deprived of his or her liberty. The court ruled that the Tribunal does not have jurisdiction to consider the legality of conditions of the CTO (and also has no jurisdiction over the treatment and detention in hospital), although this may be relevant in deciding whether statutory criteria for the CTO are met. However, 'if the tribunal identifies a state of affairs amounting to an unlawful deprivation of liberty, it must be within its powers to explain to all concerned what the true legal effect of a CTO is'. If the patient wishes to challenge his unlawful deprivation of liberty under the CTO, other than by periodic applications to the Tribunal, the legal remedy is through habeas corpus or judicial review.

What Happens if the Patient Breaks a Condition?

If a patient doesn't adhere to a condition, there are a number of options open to the Responsible Clinician. These include changing the conditions or discharging the patient from the CTO. It may be that the patient's circumstances have changed or their health improved and the condition is no longer necessary. However, given that the conditions were necessary to minimise risk, a patient's failure to comply means that serious consideration should be given to recalling them to hospital. This highlights the import-ance of always discussing with the patient, carers, if relevant, and the supervising team what conditions should be placed on the patient. For example, it might be a lawful condition for the patient to avoid alcohol or illicit drugs. But if abstinence is to be made a condition, there must be a plan as to how this is to be monitored and what action would be taken if the patient transgresses – perhaps even slightly.

The patient may appeal against a CTO (but not against its conditions) to the Hospital Managers or the Tribunal. If a patient has lodged an appeal against their detention order and, while waiting for the hearing, is placed on a CTO, the Tribunal will go ahead as planned, as a CTO Tribunal, i.e. the patient isn't required to put in a fresh application.

Discharge from a CTO

It may seem self-evident that once the patient is well, and no longer meets the criteria for a CTO, then the patient must be discharged. However, we know that the current discharge rate by both Responsible Clinicians and the Tribunal from CTOs is very low. Patients are staying on them for a long time. The Tribunal discharge rate from a CTO remains less than for detained patients. It is argued that this is because the criteria for a CTO are so wide.[5]

One way to look at it is that if the patient remains ill, then the CTO is clearly still required. Equally, if the patient is now well and complying with medication and conditions, then the CTO is working and, therefore, still appropriate. It is important to remember that CTOs have an impact on a person's autonomy. Getting the balance right, between the risks of a relapse, with serious consequences for the patient and/or others, and overriding the patient's right to self-determination isn't easy.

Exactly the same people may discharge a patient from a CTO as from detention, i.e. the Responsible Clinician, the Nearest Relative (but subject to a barring order from the Responsible Clinician), the Hospital Managers and the Tribunal.

A question that has arisen in relation to discharging a CTO by the Tribunal is the degree of imminence of relapse. The case of *LW* v. *Cornwall Partnership NHS Foundation Trust*,[6] which concerned three unconnected individuals (LW, SE and TS), addressed this. The grounds for their appeal were that there should be a degree of imminence of relapse required, i.e. in the *near future*, before a person could be lawfully maintained as a community patient on a CTO. This had been successfully argued for a patient (Mr M) detained in hospital because 'there was no real evidence to support its [the Tribunal's] view that non-compliance with medication and the risk of consequent relapse *in the near future* would probably occur'.[7] However, their appeals were dismissed. 'Where there is a risk of relapse which might necessitate recall, it will be a relevant consideration when it is thought likely such a relapse will occur; but that factor is not itself determinative.' Although all relevant circumstances must be considered, there is no requirement 'as a matter of law that likely relapse must be "soon", "in the near future" or within the permitted duration of a CTO for discharge to be lawfully refused'.

Renewal of a CTO

If all is going well, but the patient continues to meet the criteria for a CTO, then it can be renewed by the Responsible Clinician with the Approved Mental Health Professional. While on a CTO, the patient may have informal admissions to hospital. Following each renewal (as for patients on a section 3, at 6 months, then a further 6 months, then annually), the patient is entitled to a further Tribunal hearing.

> **Note**
> Patients subject to a CTO may be admitted to hospital informally, i.e. while remaining on their CTO. There is, however, a potential difficulty. Section 5 cannot be applied to an informally admitted CTO patient. In other words, the only option to prevent the patient leaving the hospital against medical advice is for the Responsible Clinician to recall the patient. This might present a problem if the Responsible Clinician is not immediately available.

Recall from a CTO

If the patient becomes unwell, or breaks one or more of the conditions, consideration will need to be given to recalling the patient to hospital.

Only the patient's Responsible Clinician has the authority to recall the patient. The recall must be in writing (form CTO3). If the letter is handed to the patient, the patient must immediately return to hospital and is considered to be AWOL until back in hospital. If it is put through the letterbox of the patient's last-known address, the patient is AWOL from just past midnight (i.e. the start of the next day). If it is posted to the patient by first-class post, the patient is AWOL from the second working day after posting. A CTO patient who is in hospital informally may be 'formally' recalled for assessment, if necessary, in that hospital or another. A patient may be recalled to any appropriate hospital (remembering the broad definition of a hospital) – it doesn't have to be the hospital responsible for the CTO.

Recall lasts up to 72 hours (from when the patient returns to hospital). There is no requirement for the patient to be admitted to a hospital bed, although this may be necessary to give sufficient time to assess, with the patient and others, what has gone wrong and the steps that need to be taken. The CTO continues to run. The Responsible Clinician can cancel the recall at any time. The rules relating to giving medical treatment to recalled patients are discussed in Chapter 8.

The MHA gives these responsibilities, which cannot be delegated, to the Responsible Clinician. Identifying the Responsible Clinician for a recalled patient should be easy but often isn't, because of the in-patient/community split and out-of-hours issues. It is essential to identify the Responsible Clinician. The Responsible Clinician who recalls the patient may not be the Responsible Clinician who authorised the patient's release, if the patient's care has been transferred following recall (e.g. from the community Responsible Clinician to an in-patient Responsible Clinician).

Patients subject to a CTO should be recalled, if necessary, rather than being detained on a section 2 or 3. If the patient, perhaps because it was not known that they were on a CTO, is detained on a section 2, the CTO continues. If the patient is detained on a section 3, the CTO is cancelled.

Revocation of a CTO

If a period in hospital exceeding 72 hours is required, and the patient again meets the criteria for detention under a treatment order, then the CTO may be revoked. The term is sometimes misunderstood. Revoking a CTO means that the patient is back on their original section – it does not mean that the patient is discharged from compulsion. This is because, as explained above, when the CTO is revoked, the underlying section, which has continued to run the whole time, comes again to the fore.

The revocation is authorised by the Responsible Clinician and an Approved Mental Health Professional. When returned to the original section (e.g. section 3 or 37), the section starts again, i.e. the patient is detained for a further 6 months. Indeed, every time a patient is placed on a CTO or the CTO is revoked, the time starts afresh. The Hospital Managers are required to refer a patient to the Tribunal as soon as practicable after revocation.

The Mental Health Act: Part IV (Consent to Treatment)

This isn't an easy topic. Common law, the Mental Capacity Act, the Mental Health Act, judicial interpretation of both, the European Convention on Human Rights and judgments of the European Court of Human Rights are all relevant. Is the treatment for mental disorder, physical disorder or both? If it is for physical illness, is the illness related in some way to the patient's mental disorder? Is the patient detained under the MHA and, if so, is it a section to which the consent to treatment provisions of the Act apply? Is the patient subject to a Community Treatment Order (CTO), in hospital or in the community, on section 17 leave or conditional discharge? What form of treatment are you considering? How old is your patient, are they competent and/or do they retain decision-making capacity? All of these questions need to be answered in order to decide whether or not the treatment can be given. It is important to remember that, if possible, the consent of the patient should always be sought, even if it isn't required.

The authority to give medical treatment for a mental disorder to a patient who is detained under the MHA or on a CTO comes from Part IV of the Act, which is entitled 'Consent to treatment'. Alas, even the nomenclature is difficult here: Part IV is divided into a Part 4 [sic] for detained patients and a Part 4A for patients on a CTO.

If the patient is informal, or detained under a section to which Part IV does not apply, or the treatment is for a physical illness unrelated to their mental disorder, then the same rules apply as for the rest of medicine – capacitous consent or use of the MCA, as discussed in Chapter 3. It is hard to understand Mr Justice Mostyn's statement in the well-publicised case of an Italian woman living in the United Kingdom who underwent a forced Caesarean section: 'I am struggling to envisage a circumstance where a patient detained under section 3 as an inpatient with a diagnosed mental illness has got capacity. It is possible, but I am struggling to imagine how it could happen.'[1] First, as previously discussed, capacity is decision specific. Second, patients almost always have capacity in relation to a large number of matters, such as what they wish to eat or wear. Third, many patients detained under section 3 are treated with their capacitous consent for both mental and physical illnesses. You should never make assumptions about a patient's capacity to make a medical decision solely on the basis of the fact that they are detained under the MHA.

Medical Treatment for Patients Detained under the MHA on Sections to which Part IV Applies

Section 56 states that all detained patients are subject to Part IV except patients detained under the very short sections, i.e. sections 4, 5(2), 5(4), 35, 135 and 136, or certain 'forensic' sections, i.e. sections 37(4), 45A(5), 73 and 74 (if the patient has not been recalled to hospital). Patients on CTOs who are recalled are included.

It is important to recognise that Part IV either applies to a particular detention section or it doesn't. There is no detention order to which Part IV partially applies. That is why, despite gossip to the contrary, there is no difference between section 2 and section 3 in relation to consent to treatment: Part IV applies to both sections.

> **Note**
> A reminder – 'medical treatment' includes nursing, psychological intervention, and specialist mental health habilitation, rehabilitation and care.

Medical Treatment for Mental Disorder

Since the court case *B* v. *Croydon Health Authority*[2] (which we discuss in Chapter 1, 'Interpretation of the MHA'), medical treatment that is for the causes or consequences of mental disorder is deemed to be treatment for mental disorder. Further, since 2007, the MHA has included the statement: 'Any reference in this Act to medical treatment, in relation to mental disorder, shall be construed as a reference to medical treatment the purpose of which is to alleviate, or prevent a worsening of, the disorder or one or more of its symptoms or manifestations.'

Therefore, a clinician can treat, without the patient's consent, a physical illness that is causing a mental disorder. A commonly asked question is whether or not self-harm resulting from mental disorder can be treated without consent. For example, may acetylcysteine be given to a detained patient who has taken an overdose of paracetamol? In a recent judgment[3] about a man with a personality disorder, Mr C, who had cut his brachial artery and kept reopening the wound, the judge said:

> It cannot be disputed that the act of self-harming, the slashing open of the brachial artery, is a symptom or manifestation of the underlying personality disorder. Therefore to treat the wound in any way is to treat the manifestation or symptom of the underlying disorder. So, indisputably, to suture the wound would be squarely within section 63. As would be the administration of a course of antibiotics to prevent infection. A consequence of bleeding from the wound is that haemoglobin levels are lowered. While it is strictly true . . . that 'low haemoglobin is not wholly a manifestation or symptom of personality disorder', it is my view that to treat the low haemoglobin by a blood transfusion is just as much a treatment of a symptom or manifestation of the disorder as is to stitch up the wound or to administer antibiotics.

So the answer is clearly yes. However, cases such as that of Mr C, where there has been a decision *not* to impose potentially life-saving treatment under section 63, should be brought before the court. This has been the case when options appear to have been exhausted and clinical teams have not wished to force nasogastric feeding on patients with intractable anorexia nervosa. As the effect of these decisions would prove potentially life-threatening, a 'full merits review'[4] undertaken by the court has been warranted in deciding that treatment should not be imposed. There are numerous cases where the courts have dealt with the issue of anorexia nervosa. Most recently, there are the cases of Ms D[5] and Ms R.[6]

Medical investigations that are required in order to give the patient medication for treating mental disorder (e.g. blood tests may be carried out if lithium or clozapine are prescribed) are also included. It is important to note that the patient must be detained under a section to which Part 4 of the MHA applies (e.g. section 2 or 3) and the 'physical' treatment must be for the cause or consequence of the mental disorder.

The courts have also ruled that there is no difference between investigations into and treatment of mental disorder.[7] A doctor had sought the High Court's permission to undertake computerised tomography of a patient (with schizophrenia and a suspected brain tumour) who refused. The judge said that there is 'no distinction between diagnostic and therapeutic procedures. The same criterion governs their lawfulness'.

There is no golden rule that says that any intervention can or can't be made using the authority of Part IV of the MHA. The circumstances of the particular case will determine the lawfulness or otherwise. A recent case does seem to stretch the notion of what may be considered medical treatment for mental disorder. In the case in question, the issue was whether haemodialysis could be medical treatment for personality disorder for the purposes of section 63.[8] The judge held that it was. The only applicable general rule is: if in doubt, seek guidance from a senior colleague or a lawyer.

Treatment for Physical Illness Unrelated to Mental Disorder

There was an important case of a patient in a high-secure hospital who developed gangrene of his leg secondary to chronic diabetes.[9] The surgeon advised that the patient would die if his leg was not amputated. The patient, who believed himself to be a doctor of international eminence (this was a delusion), refused surgery, saying he had complete confidence that God and the hospital staff would save him. He accepted that it was possible he would die from the gangrene, but remained adamant he did not want surgery. The case went to court. The judge said that the physical disorder, the gangrene, was unrelated to the patient's mental disorder and the patient's refusal was not part of, or related to, his psychotic thinking and therefore the MHA was not relevant. Furthermore, the patient was able to understand, remember, believe and weigh the information in the balance in order to make a decision and express that decision. (Although the case pre-dated the MCA, the rules relating to incapacity were almost identical to current rules, except that 'believe' has been removed as it was thought to be unnecessary – it is subsumed within 'weigh in the balance'.) The patient was deemed to have capacity to make the decision and refuse the surgery. He, and his leg, recovered. Some people, including his own solicitor, have questioned whether or not he did have capacity. Remembering that it was assumed that the patient was going to die, his solicitor thought she ought to discuss with him the making of a will. He thought that this was a good idea (he had quite a lot of money as he had not spent any of his benefit in the 30 or so years he had been in Broadmoor). He said that he wanted to leave the money to himself as he would need it after he had died!

Along with many others, we think that, had the patient injured his leg as an act of self-harm due to his schizophrenia, then the leg could, lawfully, have been amputated.

Caesarean Section without Consent

A number of judgments have been handed down regarding pregnant women who may lack capacity to make decisions regarding their obstetric care because of mental disorder.

In two early cases, the MHA was used to force a Caesarean section on women who, for differing reasons, refused to consent. These are not to be confused with the often-quoted case of the woman who consented to a Caesarean section, but refused at the last moment because she had a 'needle phobia':[10] the MHA was not relevant in that case.

One of the cases[11] concerned a woman suffering from schizophrenia detained under section 3. The court decided that the Caesarean section was 'ancillary' (see Chapter 1, 'Interpretation of the MHA') to the treatment of her mental disorder because:

- it would prevent a deterioration in the patient's mental state;
- for the successful treatment of the patient's schizophrenia, it was necessary for her to give birth to a live child;
- the administration of antipsychotic drugs had been necessarily interrupted by pregnancy and could not be resumed until the child was born.

The Caesarean was lawful under section 63. To explain the marked contrast in the decision in this case from that in *Re. C*, the judge said that: 'Treatment of C's gangrene was not likely to affect his mental condition.'[12] Given that it was thought that C would die without the surgery, we find this rather odd.

In the other case,[13] a woman with pre-eclampsia who refused a Caesarean section was detained under the MHA for assessment of her mental state. A Court authorisation for the Caesarean section was then sought and obtained. Following successful delivery of the baby, the patient was discharged from hospital. The patient complained that the Caesarean section had been carried out unlawfully (despite the court authorisation). The Court of Appeal said that the patient was unlawfully detained. Although she may have had a mental disorder, this was clearly not the reason for her detention because she was neither assessed nor treated for her mental disorder. The judicial authority for the Caesarean section had been based on false and incomplete information. The court repeated that a competent pregnant woman can refuse treatment even if that refusal may result in harm to her or her unborn child, i.e. the unborn child does not have a legal existence other than as part of its mother.

More recently, in a judgment regarding a woman with schizoaffective disorder detained under the MHA, detailed guidance was provided as to why and when an application to court should be made for a pregnant woman who lacks, or may lack, capacity.[14] The judge confirmed the above guidance, saying 'in appropriate circumstances s 63 MHA may authorise medical treatment when the primary purpose of the same is to alleviate or prevent a worsening in P's psychiatric illness or its symptoms. If obstetric treatment can be provided under s 63, it can be performed without P's consent using proportionate and necessary restraint'.

The judge went on to point out that (bearing in mind the presumption of capacity even when patients are detained under the MHA) where capacity is lacking, 'in the vast majority of these cases obstetric care will be provided to P under the MCA with the powers under the MHA being used to facilitate P receiving that care at an acute hospital under the MCA'. Furthermore, any deprivation of liberty will need to be appropriately authorised. However, there are circumstances when application to court should be made:

- the interventions proposed probably amount to serious medical treatment;
- there is a real risk that the person will be subject to more than transient forcible restraint;
- there is a serious dispute as to what obstetric care is in her best interests;

- there is a real risk that the person will suffer a deprivation of her liberty which cannot be authorised under the MCA;
- where delivery by Caesarean section is proposed and the merits of the proposal are finely balanced or delivery by Caesarean section is likely to involve more than transient forcible restraint.

This is one sphere, and there are others, to which we alluded in Chapter 1 where clinicians should be mindful of the exceptional nature of the decisions to be made. Thereby consider, first, should an application to court be made and then how soon should it be made? Trusts have attracted criticism by submitting avoidably late applications.[15]

Treatment Groups under the MHA

There are five different groups of treatments under the MHA:

1. treatments that always require *both* the patient's capacitous consent *and* a statutory second opinion (section 57); the rules for this group of interventions apply to informal patients as well as to detained ones;
2. treatments that always *either* require capacitous consent *or* a statutory second opinion and which cannot be given in the face of capacitous refusal (except in an emergency) (section 58A);
3. treatments that, 3 months or more after first being given during the detention, require either the capacitous consent of the patient (certified by the Responsible Clinician or Approved Clinician in charge of that treatment) or a statutory second opinion (section 58); these treatments may, for the first 3 months, be given under the authority of section 63 – see below;
4. treatments that can always be given on the authority of the Responsible Clinician (or, when appropriate, the Approved Clinician in charge of that treatment) (section 63);
5. emergency ('urgent') treatments (section 62).

The Secretary of State for Health has the authority to add, or remove, treatments from each category as he or she thinks appropriate. The surgical implantation of hormones for the purpose of reducing male sex drive was added to the first category (section 57) in this way. There has been a great deal of discussion as to whether or not forced tube-feeding for mental disorder (anorexia nervosa) should be added to group 3 (section 58). To date, this has not been done.

Section 57 – Treatment Requiring Consent and a Second Opinion

The two treatments that always require the capacitous consent of patients (both formal and detained) and a statutory second opinion are:

- psychosurgery for mental disorder;
- the surgical implantation of hormones for the purpose of reducing male sex drive.

The statutory second opinion is from a three-person team, two of whom are non-medical, whose role is to confirm that the patient is capacitous and consenting, and a Second Opinion Appointed Doctor (SOAD).

Section 58A – Electroconvulsive Therapy

Electroconvulsive therapy (ECT) for mental disorder always requires *either* capacitous consent *or* a SOAD and cannot be given in the face of capacitous refusal (except in an emergency).

- Other than in an emergency, ECT cannot be given to a capacitous patient who refuses it. Further, it cannot be given to an incapacitous patient who has made a valid applicable advance refusal, or if a health and welfare attorney or a court or a court deputy refuses to permit the treatment.
- ECT can be given as urgent treatment (under section 62) to a capacitous patient who is refusing, or in the face of a valid applicable advance refusal, or where a health and welfare attorney or a court or court deputy refuses to permit the treatment, but only for two of the four 'urgent treatment' grounds, i.e.:
  - treatment that is immediately necessary to save the patients' life; or
  - treatment (not being irreversible) that is immediately necessary to prevent a deterioration in his condition.

  Whether these grounds are ever likely to be fulfilled for a capacitous patient is a moot point.
- There is no set number of ECT treatments that can be given in an emergency. It can continue so long as the treatment is required as an emergency on the grounds above. A SOAD is not required, nor is there any purpose in asking for one, because a SOAD certificate cannot override capacitous refusal. Once the emergency has ended, the ECT must be stopped unless the patient is now consenting. This applies even if it means that the patient may relapse and again need ECT as an emergency.
- The authority to prescribe ECT comes from the Responsible Clinician's certificate (or, when appropriate, the certificate of the Approved Clinician in charge of ECT) or the SOAD's certificate.
  - If the patient is capacitous and consenting, as assessed by the Responsible Clinician (or Approved Clinician in charge of ECT), this must be recorded in the patient's medical record and the appropriate form completed. The form should specify the maximum number of treatments to which the patient has consented.
  - If the patient lacks capacity to consent, a SOAD certificate is required. This is requested by the patient's Responsible Clinician (or Approved Clinician in charge of the treatment). The request must include a clear, written treatment plan for the patient. The SOAD must examine the patient and consult two people who have been professionally concerned with the patient's medical treatment. One of the two consultees must be a nurse and the other neither a nurse nor a Registered Medical Practitioner. The patient's Responsible Clinician cannot be a consultee, but the SOAD is expected to discuss the case with the Responsible Clinician. Only then may the SOAD issue a certificate (assuming the SOAD confirms the appropriateness of ECT).
  - A SOAD certificate plus the patient's consent (if capacitous) or consent from a parent or guardian (if lacking competence) is required if ECT is to be given to a minor.

Section 58 – Treatment Requiring Consent or a Second Opinion

Section 58(1)(b) applies to:

> The administration of medicine to a patient by any means ... at any time during a period for which he is liable to be detained as a patient to whom this Part of this Act applies if three months or more have elapsed since the first occasion in that period when medicine was administered to him by any means for his mental disorder. [i.e. to medication for mental disorder after 3 months]

The authority for the first 3 months of medication comes from section 63. This is known as the 3-month rule.

- What this means is that 3 months after the first dose of medication for mental disorder is given, within a continuous period of detention, either the capacitous consent of the patient or a SOAD certificate is required.
- The 3-months clock starts ticking only when Part IV of the Act applies: medication given while the patient is detained under section 5 doesn't count. If a patient is detained under section 4, the clock ticks from the start if the section 4 is converted to a section 2 (because the start of the section 2 is backdated to the start of the section 4), but if the patient is put on a section 3 directly from the section 4, then the clock doesn't start until the start of the section 3 (because Part IV doesn't apply to section 4 patients).
- If a patient is detained but doesn't receive medication for mental disorder straight away, then the clock doesn't tick until medication is given.
- It makes no difference if a single dose of medication is given on admission and then no more is given for weeks. The clock has started.
- At the end of the 3-month period, medication for mental disorder can be lawfully given to a detained patient only with the authority of a certificate (unless given as urgent treatment under section 62).

Authority for Capacitous Consenting Patients

- If the patient is capacitous and consenting, the certificate of authority is completed by the Responsible Clinician, unless the Responsible Clinician is not suitably qualified (i.e. is neither a Registered Medical Practitioner nor a nurse prescriber). In such a case, the certificate must be completed by the Approved Clinician in charge of medication.
- The Responsible Clinician (or Approved Clinician in charge) should record in the patient's medical record the assessment of the patient's capacity and consent.
- The information on the certificate should include:
  . the medication by *British National Formulary* (BNF) category;
  . the maximum number of drugs from each category;
  . the maximum dose of each drug or category (this can be done either by quantity, e.g. 300 mg, or by reference to the BNF dose range, e.g. 'within BNF dose range' or 'up to one-and-a-half times maximum BNF dose'); if more than one drug in a particular category is authorised, the form should specify whether the maximum is per drug or per category;
  . the route, or routes, of administration (e.g. oral or intramuscular).

Authority for Capacitous Refusing or Incapacitous Patients

- If the patient is capacitous and refusing or lacks capacity, a SOAD certificate is required. The SOAD procedure is the same as for ECT above.

  . The SOAD is not obliged to agree with the Responsible Clinician's plan (or the role would be pointless!). The SOAD may amend the plan as he or she thinks appropriate. This should be done in discussion with the Responsible Clinician. The final decision rests with the SOAD. There is no appeal against the decision of a SOAD.
  . The SOAD certificate should be detailed in the same way as the Responsible Clinician's certificate.
  . The SOAD certificate may be time limited.

- Patients on conditional discharge (from a section 37 with a section 41 restriction order) are not subject to Part IV of the MHA. The 3-month rule starts again if such a patient is recalled to hospital.

Placebo Medication (for Mental Disorder)

Can patients subject to the MHA be given placebo medication for their mental disorder? One dictionary definition of placebo is 'a substance given to someone who is told that it is a particular medicine ...' (http://dictionary.cambridge.org). Another, 'a substance that is administered as a drug but has no medicinal content ...' (www .chambersharrap.co.uk).

One side of the argument says that a placebo isn't medication. If this is the case, section 58 is irrelevant, and the placebo is a treatment under section 63 which doesn't require the patient's consent (although the MHA Code of Practice says that 'the patient's consent should still be sought').[16] The alternative point of view is that it is medication as far as the patient is concerned. This means that it needs to be discussed properly with the patient in order to determine whether or not the patient is capacitous and consenting – which is obviously self-defeating.

Covert Medication (for Mental Disorder)

Unlike a placebo, covert medication is medication. Its use, therefore, is subject to section 63 for the first 3 months and section 58 thereafter. It is again difficult to see how one can assess whether or not the patient is capacitous and consenting without discussing the medication with them. There is an additional difficulty with covert medication. A patient whose condition improves as a result of covert medication will presume that they have got better without medication. Should the patient appeal against their section to a Tribunal (or Hospital Managers), they would be in an impossible position. They would, entirely reasonably, argue that they didn't need medication. The Responsible Clinician would have to explain why this wasn't true. The Upper Tribunal has established that this information (that the patient is being given covert medication) cannot be withheld from the patient if they have made a Tribunal appeal[17] (although we are aware that, despite this ruling, many Tribunals do agree to the information being kept from the patient).

Notes

- All prescribed medication for mental disorder, including 'as required' (prn) medication, should be authorised by the Responsible Clinician's or SOAD's certificate.
- Medication that is not for mental disorder should not be on the certificate. So, for example, sodium valproate prescribed as a mood stabiliser should be included, whereas sodium valproate prescribed for epilepsy should not be.
- Just what should be included on the certificate isn't always clear or logical. The Care Quality Commission (CQC) states that anticholinergics prescribed for the adverse effects of antipsychotics should be authorised on the certificate, but laxatives prescribed for the adverse effects of antipsychotics should not be.[18]
- It is the certificate itself that authorises the treatment.

A Legal Problem with Section 58

There is a legal difficulty in relation to section 58 treatments for which we don't have an answer (other than to say that we are not aware of any relevant case law). The Act states (section 58(3)(a)) that, other than in relation to section 62 (i.e. urgent treatment):

> a patient shall not be given any form of treatment to which this section applies unless:
>
> (a) he has consented to that treatment and either the approved clinician in charge of it or a registered medical practitioner appointed for the purposes of this Part of this Act by the regulatory authority has certified in writing that the patient is capable of understanding its nature, purpose and likely effects and has consented to it . . .

So, if the patient is capacitous and consenting, the Responsible Clinician (or Approved Clinician in charge of medication) will have completed the required certificate (in England, form T2; in Wales, form CO 2) and that gives the authority to treat the patient. But what about out-of-hours? At these times, the duty consultant becomes the Responsible Clinician (or Approved Clinician in charge of medication). The Codes of Practice (England and Wales), when describing the circumstances in which certificates cease to authorise treatment, state that for certificates issued by an Approved Clinician under section 58 or 58A: 'The clinician concerned stops being the approved clinician in charge of the treatment.' This suggests that either the patient is examined and a new form is completed every 8 hours or so, or the patient should not be given medication for mental disorder out-of-hours (other than under section 62). The Care Quality Commission has recognised this difficulty and gives the following advice:

> The person who is the 'approved clinician in charge of the treatment in question' is a question of fact, and the role may pass from one clinician to another frequently during a patient's detention in hospital. This can be because the patient moves to a different ward or security level; because clinicians leave or enter employment with the detaining authority, or their responsibilities are reorganised; or simply as a result of a clinician taking leave or being otherwise unavailable to fulfil the role.
>
> It is impractical of the law to require re-certification of the patient's capacity and consent in all these circumstances. Where a clinician is only fulfilling the role temporarily, it appears to be unnecessarily bureaucratic. Also, requiring re-certification before any routine treatment may be counter-productive in terms of a safeguard for patients, as it could encourage clinicians to 'rubber-stamp' certificates without spending an appropriate time to

review the medication, and personally check that the patient is giving informed consent and has the capacity to do so.

Some legal commentators have suggested that the interpretation of the revised Code on this matter is open to doubt. Detaining authorities may choose to disregard the Code's advice on such grounds, and on the impracticality of following it to the letter. We hope that, if they do disregard the advice, they will continue to require that a new form T2 is completed when there is a permanent change of approved clinician in charge of the treatment ... even if they allow (as has been common practice for many years) a 'hand-over' period. In these circumstances, we take the view that the old form continues to be the authorising treatment until the new clinician has had time to speak with the patient and assess whether re-certification is appropriate.[19]

> **Note**
> It is important to remember that patients who are being treated with their consent under section 57 or 58 can withdraw their consent at any time (section 60) and that if they do so, then the treatment must stop unless the provisions of section 62 below are met.

Section 62 – Urgent Treatment

Compliance with sections 58 and 58A is not required if the treatment meets the description of 'urgent treatment'. 'Urgent treatment' can be authorised by any Registered Medical Practitioner or an Approved Clinician who is a nurse prescriber. There are four categories of 'urgent treatment' (only the first two apply to ECT). 'Urgent treatment' is treatment that is:

- immediately necessary to save a patient's life; or
- immediately necessary (and not irreversible) to prevent a serious deterioration in the patient's condition; or
- immediately necessary (and neither irreversible nor hazardous) to alleviate serious suffering; or
- immediately necessary (and neither irreversible nor hazardous) and the minimum interference required to prevent the patient from behaving violently or being a danger to themselves or others.

What is meant by irreversible and hazardous isn't made entirely clear, even though they are defined: 'For the purposes of this section treatment is irreversible if it has unfavourable irreversible physical or psychological consequences and hazardous if it entails significant physical hazard.'

In addition, if a capacitous patient has been consenting to medication and then withdraws consent, the patient may be required to continue with the medication if stopping 'would cause serious suffering to the patient'.

There is no statutory form for section 62 treatments. Most hospitals have their own form.

Section 63 – Treatment Not Requiring Consent

This section applies to treatments that can always be given on the authority of the Responsible Clinician (or Approved Clinician in charge of that treatment) and for which the patient's consent is not required (this does not mean that consent shouldn't, if possible, be sought). These include any medical treatment (remember the broad definition given in Chapter 5, 'Medical Treatment') not covered by section 57 or 58 (including 58A) above. It covers not only nursing, psychological treatments and so on, but also medication for mental disorder for the first 3 months (section 58 applies only after 3 months).

Common Mistakes after the 3-Month Rule

- A patient being treated for schizophrenia requests an antidepressant. The Responsible Clinician agrees. It's prescribed. No one thinks about the certificate requirements.
- A patient is being prescribed an oral antipsychotic. Following discussion, it is agreed to start a depot. The certificate doesn't authorise depot administration, but this has been forgotten.
- A patient requests a sleeping tablet. The duty doctor interviews the patient, who is clearly capacitous and consenting. The doctor prescribes the medication, but it isn't authorised on the certificate. Only the Responsible Clinician (or Approved Clinician in charge of medication) is deemed able to assess a patient's capacity and consent and to complete the authorisation.
- The team doctor prescribes 'as required' (prn) medication. The certificate authorises one antipsychotic. The doctor has just prescribed another. Or, although two are authorised, the total dose now goes above that which is authorised. Or, the certificate authorised the administration of the antipsychotic orally and the doctor has just prescribed that it may be given intramuscularly.
- The authorising certificate is completed by the Responsible Clinician, i.e. it is confirming that the patient is capacitous and consenting. The patient refuses the medication and the 'as required' (prn), authorised on the form, is forced on the patient.

> **Important**
> Medication for mental disorder, after 3 months, can only be given lawfully if it is authorised on the appropriate form or identified as being given as an emergency under section 62. Medication given outside these parameters is an assault.

Community Treatment Orders and Consent to Treatment (under Part 4A: Treatment of Community Patients Not Recalled to Hospital)

Unfortunately, the consent to treatment provisions in relation to CTO patients, be they in the community, recalled or following revocation of the CTO, are very complex.

Part 4 does not apply while patients are in the community, hence the addition of Part 4A in 2007. If the patient is recalled to hospital, Part 4 applies with modifications. If the CTO is revoked, Part 4 applies and Part 4A doesn't (with one exception).

> **Note**
> The certificate requirements for CTO patients who are capacitous and consenting have been changed by the Health and Social Care Act 2012.

Rules in Relation to CTO Patients in the Community

There are two requirements for CTO patients in the community to be given medication for mental disorder. These are:

- the usual authority: this is the same as would be required to give a patient medication if they were not subject to the MHA, i.e.:
  - . the patient's consent if the patient has capacity; or
  - . in the patient's best interest if the patient lacks capacity, *but* only if the patient does not resist or it is given with the authority of a person with a lasting power of attorney for health and welfare decisions (and the decision comes within the scope of that authority); also, there must not be an advance refusal or refusal by the attorney or court;

- a certificate: the Part 4A certificate is signed by the Responsible Clinician (or Approved Clinician with responsibility for medication) if the patient has capacity and is consenting; the certificate is signed by a SOAD if the patient lacks capacity.

So, while informal patients may be treated solely with the appropriate authorisation, CTO patients also require a certificate.

> **Note**
> The certificate requirement does not apply for the first month of the CTO or for the first 3 months since the start of the detention, whichever is later.

- Capacitous consenting CTO patients can be given medication for mental disorder that is not on the Part 4A Responsible Clinician (or Approved Clinician with responsibility for medication) certificate only in an emergency and with the patient's consent. If they do not consent, capacitous CTO patients in the community cannot be forced to take medication for mental disorder even in an emergency. Capacitous CTO patients can at any time withdraw their consent to take medication.
- Capacitous consenting CTO patients taking medication for mental disorder authorised by the Responsible Clinician (or Approved Clinician with responsibility for medication) who lose capacity will require a SOAD certificate if they are to continue taking that medication. The medication can continue while waiting for the SOAD authorisation if the Responsible Clinician (or Approved Clinician with responsibility for medication) believes that stopping it will cause the patient serious suffering.
- Incapacitous CTO patients cannot be prescribed medication for mental disorder, even if it is included on the Part 4A SOAD certificate, if there is a valid advance refusal/power of attorney/court order refusing such medication or the patient is refusing or resisting taking it.
- Incapacitous CTO patients may be given medication for mental disorder that is not SOAD certified in an emergency, under section 64, using proportionate force as necessary.

Although the 3-month rule applies, i.e. if the patient is placed on a CTO during the first 3 months of detention there are no certificate requirements governing medication for mental disorder, the situation is not quite the same as it is for detained patients, because community patients can't generally be forced to have treatment (this is explained further below).

No matter how long the patient has been detained, there are no certificate requirements for the first month as a CTO patient. Within that month, a certificate must be obtained if the patient is to continue to be prescribed medication for mental disorder thereafter. If the patient is capacitous and consenting, it is a Responsible Clinician (or Approved Clinician with responsibility for medication) certificate. If the patient lacks capacity, it is a SOAD certificate. The SOAD certificate must specify whether the authorised medication can be given only with incapacitous compliance or whether it can also be given, in whole or in part, following recall, despite the patient's objection. Unlike for detained patients, no certificate exists that enables medication for mental disorder to be given to a capacitous patient who refuses it while in the community, because such a patient cannot be forced to accept medication.

Rules in Relation to CTO Patients on Recall

- If it is less than a month since the start of the CTO, there are no certificate requirements.
- If it is more than a month since the start of the CTO, the patient:
  - if capacitous and consenting, can be treated with the authority of the Responsible Clinician (or Approved Clinician with responsibility for medication);
  - if capacitous but now refusing medication certified by the Responsible Clinician (or Approved Clinician with responsibility for medication), can only be required to take it following authorisation by a SOAD or under the 'urgent treatment' provisions of section 62;
  - if incapacitous, can be required to take medication that the Part 4A SOAD certificate has specified can be given in this circumstance and can be given urgent medication under the provisions of section 62.

Rules Following Revocation of the CTO

- The patient is detained and subject to Part 4 of the MHA. Medication for mental disorder must be authorised either by the Responsible Clinician (or Approved Clinician in charge of the treatment) if the patient is capacitous and consenting or by a Part 4 SOAD certificate if capacitous and refusing or incapacitous.
- The patient can be treated with the authority of the SOAD Part 4A certificate if applicable and the patient has one, until a Part 4 certificate can be provided.
- The patient can be given emergency medication under section 62.

SOAD Visits

It is the Responsible Clinician's responsibility to ensure that patients are treated lawfully. This means, first, making a request to the CQC for a SOAD in plenty of time, giving at least 3 weeks' notice (for a patient on a CTO, the request should be made as soon as the CTO is applied for). Second, it means enabling the SOAD to undertake their responsibilities before they furnish a certificate. For this, the Responsible Clinician should identify the two professionals the SOAD will interview, make sure they are available for the interview and, more difficult, ensure that the patient and their clinical record are available.

The clinical record also includes electronic patient records. The two consultees, neither of whom can be the Responsible Clinician (or Approved Clinician in charge of the treatment), are 'persons who have been professionally concerned with the patient's medical treatment'. For detained patients, they will be a nurse and a professional who is neither a nurse nor a Registered Medical Practitioner; for CTO patients, they may be any professional, but only one may be a Registered Medical Practitioner.

As we mentioned in Chapter 1, SOADs are required to provide written reasons in support of their decision to approve treatment plans for patients. The MHA Code of Practice also requires that the clinician in charge of the treatment communicate the results of the SOAD visit to the patient, unless the clinician or SOAD thinks there is the likelihood of serious harm ensuing. The Care Quality Commission will expect to see evidence that this discussion has taken place (or why it has not).

Chapter 9

Appeals against Detention/ Compulsion

Rights of Appeal

Everyone deprived of their liberty must have a right of appeal. Patients detained under the MHA have two rights of appeal. They may appeal against their detention or CTO to the Hospital Managers (usually a group of people appointed for the purpose of hearing appeals) and to the First-Tier Tribunal of the Health, Education and Social Care chamber, known as the FTT, the Mental Health Tribunal or just the Tribunal. All appeals panels consist of three people.

The Hospital Managers

Hospital Managers are 'lay' people in the sense that, although they may (and usually do) have qualifications and very considerable experience in mental health, they are not appointed on the basis of specific professional requirements. Patients may appeal to the Hospital Managers whenever they wish. The appeals panel will expect written reports from the Responsible Clinician, a nurse (or the care coordinator for a patient on a CTO) and an Approved Mental Health Professional prior to the hearing. It requires three or more Hospital Managers to agree that the patient should be discharged from detention. (Although this appears to mean that they could, in theory, have a panel of seven and discharge the patient despite the majority being in favour of detention, general legal principles would make this unlawful.) The Hospital Managers are required to hold a hearing if the Responsible Clinician issues a barring order preventing the patient's Nearest Relative from discharging the section. Under this circumstance, although it is essential for the Responsible Clinician to address the issue of dangerousness at the hearing, the Hospital Managers have an additional discretion not to discharge the patient even if they do not accept the 'dangerousness' criterion.[1] They also review all section 20 renewals and may hold a hearing if the patient contests the renewal.

Hospital Managers have responsibilities to refer a patient to the Tribunal for a hearing at defined times if the patient has not applied for one: after 6 months and then every 3 years for adults and annually for minors, and following revocation of a CTO or conditional discharge.

The guidance below, in relation to writing reports and giving evidence for Tribunals, is also appropriate for Hospital Managers' hearings.

Mental Health Tribunal

The Tribunal fulfils the European Convention on Human Rights function of a court. Each panel is chaired by a judge (a more senior judge in the case of patients on restriction orders) and has a Medical Member (a Registered Medical Practitioner) and a Specialist Member with well-founded and practical experience of working in the health and welfare fields in either the statutory, voluntary or private sector. The patient is entitled to representation by a lawyer (representation is not means tested). The panel will require reports from the Responsible Clinician, a nurse who is involved in the patient's care (or the care coordinator, for CTO patients) and an Approved Mental Health Professional and from other involved professionals as appropriate.

The Tribunal rules for Wales and for England can be found in secondary legislation.[2]

A detained or CTO patient is entitled to a Tribunal appeal once within each detention or renewal period (although there is no appeal for the first 6 months of a section 37). It must be requested within the first 14 days for section 2. Otherwise, patients may appeal once in the first 6 months, once in the second 6 months and then once a year. Patients are also entitled to a Tribunal hearing each time they are placed on a CTO or a CTO is revoked.

The Nearest Relative may request a Tribunal if the Responsible Clinician has barred the Nearest Relative's request for discharge of a patient on a section 3. In addition, the Hospital Managers must refer the patient to a Tribunal if the patient has not had a Tribunal hearing after the first 6 months of detention or within 3 years thereafter.

There are often delays between an application or reference being made to the Tribunal and the hearing itself. What if there is a change in the individual's legal status in the meantime? If a patient on a section 2 applies for a Tribunal hearing but is placed on a section 3 before it takes place, they will be entitled to both their section 2 hearing (although to section 3 criteria) and their section 3 hearing. Similarly, if a patient is placed on a CTO while awaiting a section 3 hearing, their section 3 appeal is carried forward (but now to CTO criteria). The same applies if a patient detained under section 3 is received into guardianship by the time of the hearing (guardianship criteria are applied). The Tribunal will not have jurisdiction if an application was made when a patient detained under section 3 is subject to a hospital order (section 37) without a restriction order before the hearing.[3]

Capacity 'Tests' and the Tribunal

The theme of capacity has emerged as a thread through a number of cases in the Upper Tribunal. There have been three different decisions differentiated for which capacity may need to be assessed in relation to a patient's application to, and representation at, the Tribunal. These are as follows:

- Does the patient have the capacity to apply to a court or tribunal to challenge his or her detention in hospital?
- Does the patient have the capacity to appoint a representative for the purpose of the Tribunal?
- Does the patient have the capacity to conduct the proceedings himself?
  To make a valid application to the Tribunal, the correct test to apply is whether the patient can understand the following (see *VS* v. *St Andrews Healthcare*[4] and *SM* v. *Livewell*[5]):
  . that they are being detained against their wishes;
  . the Tribunal is a body that would be able to decide whether they should be released.

As Judge Jacobs stressed in the case of Mr S, the capacity to bring proceedings is not the same as capacity to then conduct those proceedings. The judge in a further case of Mr A[6] drew a distinction between the 'capacity to appoint a representative' and the 'capacity to conduct proceedings'. However, he indicated that this distinction 'narrows' and can be 'theoretical rather than real'. It is perhaps as well for our purposes to assume they are the same.

Tribunal rules mean that a Trust may be directed to determine whether the person is capable of conducting the proceeding. The Responsible Clinician will be requested to complete an MH3 form. If lacking the relevant decision-making capacity, the Tribunal, under rule 11(7)(b), can appoint a lawyer to act on the behalf of the patient. If capacity to conduct proceedings is in doubt, it is helpful to identify this as early as possible certainly in reports, but also through the MHA administration department.

The MH3 form asks the following questions:

- 'Does the patient lack the mental capacity to make a decision as to whether they wish to be represented before the tribunal?' Yes or no.
- 'If lacking capacity is it your assessment that it would be in the best interests of the patient to be represented?' (and provide reasons if not).
- 'In any case where you assess that the patient does have capacity to make a decision to appoint a representative, has the patient stated either that they do not wish to conduct their own case or that they wish to be represented (in either case the tribunal may appoint a representative for them)?'

Guidance on the capacity test to apply is provided on the form as follows:

'A patient who has impairment or disturbance to the functioning of his/her brain or mind probably lacks capacity to make a decision to appoint a representative if the answer is "No" to one or more of the following non-exhaustive list of questions:

(a) Does the patient understand what a tribunal hearing is?
(b) Does the patient understand what the tribunal's powers are (e.g. to discharge the Section/order)?
(c) Does the patient understand the purpose and role of the representative (e.g. to question the clinical team on the patient's behalf and tell the panel what the patient's views are)?
(d) Can the patient assess the consequences of their decision one way or the other (e.g. appreciate that if they are not represented their chances of being discharged may not be as good as they would be with a representative, because the clinical team will not be challenged and the tribunal may not know what the patient wants)?
(e) Can the patient communicate their decision sufficiently clearly to be understood?'

We have seen in Chapter 2, as in the case of Ms K,[7] where the patient lacks the capacity to make an application the case must be struck out because of non-compliance with Tribunal rules. These procedural issues can appear somewhat confusing, but staff making applications on a patient's behalf in good faith may not be acting lawfully. As things have evolved where the Tribunal forms the view that the patient never had capacity to make application, it must then strike the case out. However, the Tribunal can now ask the parties whether they would argue that it would nevertheless be in the patient's best interests to review the criteria. The Tribunal judge can then adjourn and make a reference under section 67 to the Department of Health, and it may be the case that the Tribunal can reconvene the same day.

The following outlines an alternative strategy to strike the necessary balance between rights and procedures:

Stage 1: Informing the patient and Nearest Relative of rights to apply to the Tribunal

Staff in the Trust should make every effort to help the patient (either directly or via their advocate) understand their rights in order to support the appeal against their detention. Thereafter, the process of appeal includes completion of the application form to the Tribunal by the patient, another professional that is authorised to do so or, under certain limited circumstances, the Nearest Relative. The application is then signed by the patient or someone authorised to do so making the application.

Stage 2: Assess capacity to bring proceedings

At the outset, consider the patient's capacity to bring proceedings assessed at the time of making the application. If the patient's capacity to challenge their detention and make an application is not clear, then the next step is to assess their capacity in accordance with the MCA (sections 1–3), applying the test in 'VS'. The nursing team, or advocate, can then submit the application form on the patient's behalf if deemed to have capacity.

Stage 3: Assess capacity to conduct proceedings

Review the questions posed in the MH3 form. The Tribunal will expect service users to be legally represented at hearings unless they decide to represent themselves and have capacity to do so.

Stage 4: Use of section 67

If the members of the clinical team are concerned that the patient lacks capacity to apply and feel that, nevertheless, they would benefit from a review of the criteria by the Tribunal, then consider whether the patient is due to be referred to the Tribunal, as described above. If so, then their case will be referred to the Tribunal in any event and no further action will be required. If there is no referral imminent, then it may be appropriate to contact the MHA administration team in the Trust asking that they make a request of the Department of Health and Social Care (DHSC) by setting out the reasons why it is felt appropriate that there should be tribunal proceedings. The DHSC team are then requested to make a referral to the Tribunal in accordance with section 67 of the Act. Anyone may ask the Secretary of State for Health to make a reference for any reason at any time. A similar duty rests on the Secretary of State for Justice in relation to restricted patients (section 71 of the MHA).

Stage 5: Keep capacity under review

The case of *PI* v. *West London Mental Health NHS Trust*[8] reminded us to keep capacity under review during tribunal proceedings. In that case, the patient had capacity to apply and had capacity to instruct, but owing to psychotic symptoms in the hearing, lost capacity and there was a need for the Tribunal to appoint the lawyer under Rule 11(7)(b) mid-way through the hearing.

Capacity assessments undertaken by clinicians may therefore influence the conduct of tribunal proceedings, but may also be subject to scrutiny. Therefore, demonstrating how the principles of the MCA have been followed (e.g. in how decision-making has been supported), identifying the information relevant to the decision and justifying and appropriate recording of assessments is important.

Reports

Section 2 hearings have to be organised quickly – the hearing must be held within 7 days of the request – so reports should be written as soon as practicable after the patient has appealed. Their content will, inevitably, be more limited than for section 3 or 37 reports. The section 3 report must be submitted within 3 weeks of the request from the Tribunal office (this is a legal requirement).

The Tribunal rules set out what evidence should go into the clinician's report for a 'mental health case'. The rules, reproduced below, are now much more specific concerning the clinical information that must be included in clinicians' reports.[9] This is more onerous for Responsible Clinicians (and others required to write reports for tribunals), but it has the advantage of clarity. Although it is tempting to write reports for tribunals as one does for general practitioners or other doctors, this is likely to give unnecessary detail about the patient while not sufficiently addressing the grounds for detention. Inadequate reports can cause adjournment of a tribunal and serious criticism of those responsible. Include the information required, under the appropriate headings, and the report cannot be criticised. There are different lists for detained, CTO, guardianship and conditionally discharged patients (there is also a requirement for additional information in social circumstances reports for patients under 18 years of age). Although the lists are long, apart from the need to comment on whether or not the patient would benefit from any changes to the process of the hearing, all the questions are to do with whether or not the patient meets the statutory requirements for detention, CTO, etc.

Given the time delay between the request for reports and the Tribunal hearing, it may be necessary to write an addendum to the initial report to bring it up to date.

Note

The Deputy Chamber President of the Tribunal wrote to hospital MHA administrators, saying that from May 2015, in relation to late reports:

> Our intention is to send a specific direction to the identified person who has failed to submit their report or statement, requiring that their written evidence be submitted within 7 days, with a warning that if this direction is not complied with, we will consider referring the person to the Upper Tribunal for consideration of a penalty.

This penalty can be a fine, with imprisonment in default.[10]

Sometimes reports from different members of the team disagree on whether or not the patient should continue to be detained. This is understandable and the differences will need to be explored by the Tribunal. It is much easier, and less embarrassing, if members of the team are aware of any differences before the hearing. Patients' solicitors will be delighted to exploit any evidence that team members haven't been talking to each other!

Extracts Reproduced from the Rules

The authors of reports should have personally met and be familiar with the patient. If an existing report becomes out-of-date, or if the status or the circumstances of the patient change after the reports have been written but before the tribunal hearing takes place (e.g. if a patient is discharged, or is recalled), the author of the report should then send to the tribunal an addendum addressing the up-to-date situation and, where necessary, the new applicable statutory criteria. This is to cover where the patient has moved to a section 3 from a section 2 while waiting for the section 2 hearing, or moved from a detained to a CTO status.

Each list of rules starts with the statement:

The report must be up-to-date, specifically prepared for the tribunal and have numbered paragraphs and pages. It should be signed and dated. The report should be written or counter-signed by the patient's Responsible Clinician. The sources of information for the events and incidents described must be made clear. This report should not be an addendum to (or reproduce extensive details from) previous reports, or recite medical records, but must briefly describe the patient's recent relevant medical history and current mental health presentation, and must include . . .

Regarding in-patients, the rules state that:

In all in-patient cases, except where a patient is detained under Section 2 of the Act, the Responsible Authority must send to the tribunal the required documents containing the specified information, so that they are received by the tribunal as soon as practicable and in any event within 3 weeks after the Authority made or received the application or reference. If the patient is a restricted patient, the Authority must also, at the same time, send copies of the documents to the Secretary of State (Ministry of Justice).

. . .

Where a patient is detained under Section 2 of the Act, the Responsible Authority must prepare the required documents as soon as practicable after receipt of a copy of the application or a request from the tribunal. If specified information has to be omitted because it is not available, then this should be mentioned in the statement or report. These documents must be made available to the tribunal panel and the patient's representative at least one hour before the hearing is due to start.

A Responsible Clinician's report on an in-patient must include:

a) whether there are any factors that may affect the patient's understanding or ability to cope with a hearing and whether there are any adjustments that the tribunal may consider in order to deal with the case fairly and justly;

b) details of any index offence(s) and other relevant forensic history;

c) a chronology listing the patient's previous involvement with mental health services including any admissions to, discharge from and recall to hospital;

d) reasons for any previous admission or recall to hospital;

e) the circumstances leading up to the patient's current admission to hospital;

f) whether the patient is now suffering from a mental disorder and, if so, whether a diagnosis has been made, what the diagnosis is, and why;

g) whether the patient has a learning disability and, if so, whether that disability is associated with abnormally aggressive or seriously irresponsible conduct;

h) depending upon the statutory criteria, whether any mental disorder present is of a nature or degree to warrant, or make appropriate, liability to be detained in a hospital for assessment and/or medical treatment;

i) details of any appropriate and available medical treatment prescribed, provided, offered or planned for the patient's mental disorder;

j) the strengths or positive factors relating to the patient;

k) a summary of the patient's current progress, behaviour, capacity and insight;

l) the patient's understanding of, compliance with, and likely future willingness to accept any prescribed medication or comply with any appropriate medical treatment for mental disorder that is or might be made available;

m) in the case of an eligible compliant patient who lacks capacity to agree or object to their detention or treatment, whether or not deprivation of liberty under the Mental Capacity Act 2005 (as amended) would be appropriate and less restrictive;

n) details of any incidents where the patient has harmed themselves or others, or threatened harm, or damaged property, or threatened damage;

o) whether (in Section 2 cases) detention in hospital, or (in all other cases) the provision of medical treatment in hospital, is justified or necessary in the interests of the patient's health or safety, or for the protection of others;

p) whether the patient, if discharged from hospital, would be likely to act in a manner dangerous to themselves or others;

q) whether, and if so how, any risks could be managed effectively in the community, including the use of any lawful conditions or recall powers . . .

A Responsible Clinician's report on a CTO patient must include:

a) where the patient is aged 18 or over and the case is a reference to the tribunal, whether the patient has capacity to decide whether or not to attend or be represented at a tribunal hearing;

b) whether, if there is a hearing, there are any factors that may affect the patient's understanding or ability to cope with it, and whether there are any adjustments that the tribunal may consider in order to deal with the case fairly and justly;

c) details of any index offence(s) and other relevant forensic history;

d) a chronology listing the patient's previous involvement with mental health services including any admissions to, discharge from and recall to hospital;

e) reasons for any previous admission or recall to hospital;

f) the circumstances leading up to the patient's most recent admission to hospital;

g) the circumstances leading up to the patient's discharge onto a CTO;

h) any conditions to which the patient is subject under Section 17B, and details of the patient's compliance;

i) whether the patient is now suffering from a mental disorder and, if so, what the diagnosis is and why;

j) whether the patient has a learning disability and, if so, whether that disability is associated with abnormally aggressive or seriously irresponsible conduct;

k) whether the patient has a mental disorder of a nature or degree such as to make it appropriate for the patient to receive medical treatment;

l) details of any appropriate and available medical treatment prescribed, provided, offered or planned for the patient's mental disorder;

m) the strengths or positive factors relating to the patient;

n) a summary of the patient's current progress, behaviour, capacity and insight;

o) the patient's understanding of, compliance with, and likely future willingness to accept any prescribed medication or comply with any appropriate medical treatment for mental disorder that is or might be made available;

p) details of any incidents where the patient has harmed themselves or others, or threatened harm, or damaged property, or threatened damage; [There are no items q) and r) in this list. T. Z.]

s) whether it is necessary for the patient's health or safety, or for the protection of others, that the patient should receive medical treatment and, if so, why;

t) whether the patient, if discharged from the CTO, would be likely to act in a manner dangerous to themselves or others;

u) whether, and if so how, any risks could be managed effectively in the community;

v) whether it continues to be necessary that the Responsible Clinician should be able to exercise the power of recall and, if so, why;

w) any recommendations to the tribunal, with reasons.[11]

Note

To clarify: when a CTO is revoked, there is an automatic referral ('reference'), by the Hospital Managers, to the Tribunal. This clause refers to circumstances when the patient is placed back on a CTO before the Tribunal hearing takes place. Although the final decision regarding whether or not a full hearing is to be held rests with the Tribunal, the patient may say they do not want a hearing. In that case, the 'Tribunal' would be undertaken solely on the basis of the reports. The Responsible Clinician's report must include an assessment of the patient's capacity 'to decide whether or not to attend or be represented'.

A Responsible Clinician's report on a guardianship patient must include:

a) whether there are any factors that may affect the patient's understanding or ability to cope with a hearing, and whether there are any adjustments that the tribunal may consider in order to deal with the case fairly and justly;

b) details of any index offence(s), and other relevant forensic history;

c) a chronology listing the patient's previous involvement with mental health services including any admissions to, discharge from and recall to hospital, and any previous instances of reception into guardianship;

d) the circumstances leading up to the patient's reception into guardianship;

e) any requirements to which the patient is subject under Section 8(1), and details of the patient's compliance;

f) whether the patient is now suffering from a mental disorder and, if so, what the diagnosis is and why;

g) whether the patient has a learning disability and, if so, whether that disability is associated with abnormally aggressive or seriously irresponsible conduct;

h) details of any appropriate and available medical treatment prescribed, provided, offered or planned for the patient's mental disorder;

i) the strengths or positive factors relating to the patient;

j) a summary of the patient's current progress, behaviour, capacity and insight;

k) the patient's understanding of, compliance with, and likely future willingness to accept any prescribed medication or comply with any appropriate medical treatment for mental disorder that is, or might be, made available;

l) details of any incidents where the patient has harmed themselves or others, or threatened harm, or damaged property, or threatened damage;

m) whether, and if so how, any risks could be managed effectively in the community;

n) whether it is necessary for the welfare of the patient, or for the protection of others, that the patient should remain under guardianship and, if so, why;

o) any recommendations to the tribunal, with reasons.

A Responsible Clinician's report on a conditionally discharged patient must include:

a) whether there are any factors that might affect the patient's understanding or ability to cope with a hearing, and whether there are any adjustments that the tribunal may consider in order to deal with the case fairly and justly;

b) details of the patient's index offence(s), and any other relevant forensic history;

c) details and details [sic] of the patient's relevant forensic history;

d) a chronology listing the patient's involvement with mental health services including any admissions to, discharge from and recall to hospital;

e) reasons for any previous recall following a Conditional Discharge and details of any previous failure to comply with conditions;

f) the circumstances leading up to the current Conditional Discharge;

g) any conditions currently imposed (whether by the tribunal or the Secretary of State), and the reasons why the conditions were imposed;

h) details of the patient's compliance with any current conditions;

i) whether the patient is now suffering from a mental disorder and, if so, what the diagnosis is and why;

j) whether the patient has a learning disability and, if so, whether that disability is associated with abnormally aggressive or seriously irresponsible conduct;

k) details of any legal proceedings or other arrangements relating to the patient's mental capacity, or their ability to make decisions or handle their own affairs;

l) details of any appropriate and available medical treatment prescribed, provided, offered or planned for the patient's mental disorder;

m) the strengths or positive factors relating to the patient;

n) a summary of the patient's current progress, behaviour, capacity and insight;

o) the patient's understanding of, compliance with, and likely future willingness to accept any prescribed medication or comply with any appropriate medical treatment for mental disorder;

p) details of any incidents where the patient has harmed themselves or others, or threatened harm, or damaged property, or threatened damage;

q) an assessment of the patient's prognosis, including the risk and likelihood of a recurrence or exacerbation of any mental disorder;

r) the risk and likelihood of the patient re-offending and the degree of harm to which others may be exposed if the patient does re-offend;

s) whether it is necessary for the patient's health or safety, or for the protection of others, that the patient should receive medical treatment and, if so, why;

t) whether the patient, if absolutely discharged, would be likely to act in a manner harmful to themselves or others, whether any such risks could be managed effectively in the community and, if so, how;

u) whether it continues to be appropriate for the patient to remain liable to be recalled for further medical treatment in hospital and, if so, why;

v) whether, and if so the extent to which, it is desirable to continue, vary and/or add to any conditions currently imposed;

w) any recommendations to the tribunal, with reasons.

> **Note**
>
> In addition to giving the information required in the Responsible Clinician's report, the Tribunal rules now require that, if there is no Social Supervisor, the Responsible Clinician's report should also provide the required social circumstances information.

Reports are copied to the patient and the patient's representative. A separate 'confidential' report may be written if you believe that information should not be shared with the patient because it would cause 'serious harm to the patient or other persons'[12] or comes from a third party. The 'confidential' report will still be shared with the patient's solicitor. If the solicitor thinks that the information should be made available to the patient, they can request the Tribunal to release the 'confidential' report to the patient. The presumption is for full disclosure and so it is for the detaining authority which is suggesting withholding information to make the case. In most cases, what information is to be withheld can be agreed between the patient's solicitor and the Responsible Clinician/detaining authority. The final decision as to whether or not information is withheld from the patient rests with the Tribunal, not with the Responsible Clinician. The threshold for 'serious harm', while varying from one panel to another, tends to be set high. (For the situation in Wales, see Appendix 1, section A1.8.)

The Hearing

The Responsible Clinician is required to attend the hearing or to make arrangements for a suitably senior colleague to attend on their behalf. The Responsible Clinician, or other witnesses, can be summoned by the Tribunal. The judge will introduce the panel, ask the witnesses to introduce themselves and ask the patient how they wish to be addressed.

The judge will usually then ask the Medical Member to report on their preliminary interview with the patient (the Medical Member has to examine the patient before the hearing for all section 2 hearings, but not for section 3 or 37 hearings unless requested by the patient) or will report the interview findings to the panel. The Medical Member is in the unusual position of being both a witness and a judge (with a small 'j'), and the patient and solicitor must be able to challenge the evidence given by the Medical Member to the other panel members. The Medical Member must be careful not to express an opinion in a way that suggests they have already come to a conclusion on any particular issue in the case.[13]

The judge will then ask the patient's solicitor who is to give evidence first – the patient or the Responsible Clinician. The Responsible Clinician (or representative) will be the first of the professionals to give evidence. Following this, all three members of the panel will ask questions of the Responsible Clinician, as will the patient's solicitor.

The Responsible Clinician (or representative) may be asked whether they wish to represent the detaining authority (or CTO equivalent), although such a question should not be asked at this stage as it should have been decided before the hearing. Any request for the Responsible Clinician to represent the relevant authority should be made by the authority itself. The Tribunal decides whether to allow such representation. If the Responsible Clinician represents the authority, then the Responsible Clinician is entitled to cross-examine the patient and other witnesses (subject to the agreement of the Tribunal) and may, if they wish and the hospital is willing to pay, be legally represented.

The patient's Nearest Relative, or other carers, may wish to attend. They may do so with the permission of the Tribunal. They may ask to give their evidence privately to the

Tribunal. Whether or not this is permitted is, again, a decision for the Tribunal. If observers (e.g. trainees or medical students) wish to attend, they or the Responsible Clinician should first ask the permission of the patient and their solicitor. It is helpful, although not essential, to let the hospital's MHA administrator or the Clerk to the Tribunal know in advance, as the permission of the Tribunal is also required. Although the Tribunal has the final say about the presence, or otherwise, of an observer, it is usually guided by the wishes of the patient and their solicitor. (For Wales, see Appendix 1, section A1.8.)

When all the evidence has been taken, everyone apart from the panel will leave the room so that the panel may make a decision. Although it varies between tribunals, it is usual for the patient, solicitor, nurse (or care coordinator, for CTO patients) and Responsible Clinician to be invited back to hear the decision.

It is important to recognise that, however unlikely you think it, the Tribunal may decide that the criteria for detention are not met. You must have thought about this option and have at least a rudimentary plan should the patient be discharged. In addition, for patients on section 3 or 37 you will be asked why the patient could not be managed on a CTO and, perhaps, what would need to happen for a CTO to be an option. For patients on CTOs, it is necessary to explain why the power of recall is required. One of the difficulties with CTOs is clarifying when they might end. As mentioned above, it can be argued that if the patient remains unwell, the CTO needs to continue, and if the patient is now well, then the CTO is working and needs to continue. For this reason, it is helpful to explain what it is hoped will be achieved by continuing the CTO and, therefore, what must change before the Responsible Clinician would discharge the patient. A possible timescale (e.g. the plan is for 1 year on a CTO to establish stability by regular medication, avoid admissions and help the patient achieve a fulfilling daily routine) is also useful.

Public Tribunal Hearings

It has been assumed that hearings would always be in private. This was recently challenged successfully (on the grounds of Article 6 of the European Convention on Human Rights) by Mr H, a patient detained in Broadmoor hospital.[14] The Upper Tribunal issued the following guidance:[15]

> Once the threshold tests (below) for establishing a right to a public hearing have been satisfied, article 6 of the European Convention on Human Rights (re-enforced by article 13 of the CRPD) requires that a patient should have the same or substantially equivalent right of access to a public hearing as a non-disabled person who has been deprived of his or her liberty, if this article 6 right to a public hearing is to be given proper effect. Such a right can only be denied a patient if enabling that right imposes a truly disproportionate burden on the state.

The threshold tests are:

(a) whether it is consistent with the subjective and informed wishes of the patient (assuming that he is competent to make an informed choice);

(b) whether it will have an adverse effect on his mental health in the short or long term, taking account of the views of those treating him and any other expert views;

(c) whether there are any other special factors for or against a public hearing;

(d) whether practical arrangements can be made for an open hearing without disproportionate burden on the hospital or relevant authority.

The Four Possible Outcomes to a Hearing

- Adjournment – for more information or because the necessary reports or people weren't available (sometimes including Tribunal members).
- Discharge from compulsion – for in-patients this is not the same as discharge from hospital. It may be agreed that the patient will stay in hospital informally.
- Deferred discharge – to a specified date in the future, usually a week or so away, to give time for aftercare arrangements to be made.
- Conditional discharge – this is for patients on restriction orders and it refers to discharge from detention (not from compulsion). The patient remains detained until such time as specified conditions are met. If the conditions cannot be met, the patient must continue to be detained. We have discussed the challenging issue of the discharge of restricted patients on conditions that amount to deprivation of liberty in Chapter 6. Notwithstanding, tribunals invariably attach a number of conditions to conditional discharge, including a requirement for patients to maintain contact with their mental healthcare team and to accept supervision from a social worker, Approved Mental Health Professional or probation officer (a 'social supervisor'), a psychiatrist (a 'psychiatric supervisor') or any other 'clinical supervisor'.[16] Surprisingly, there was no clear legal requirement for a medical supervisor until a particular case[17] emphasised that to recall the patient, the Secretary of State must comply with the *Winterwerp* judgment (see Chapter 2, 'Convention Articles'), i.e. there must be evidence of mental disorder determined on the basis of 'objective medical expertise'.[18] The MHA Code of Practice states that 'other than in an emergency, medical evidence will be required that the patient is currently mentally disordered'.[19]

Note

The rules in relation to restricted patients are complex and guidance, if required, should be sought from the Ministry of Justice.

Personal Thoughts on Reports and Giving Evidence

It is important, if possible, not to hurt patients' feelings or harm the relationship between the Responsible Clinician and the patient, in either written or oral evidence. To this end, we recommend the following.

- Make it clear when the information you give is what others have written in the patient's notes rather than information you have gathered directly from the patient or while the patient was under your care. Preface the former with 'It is recorded that'. If the patient has told you that the information isn't true, then (a) point out to them that it is true that it is recorded and (b) write in the report that the patient says it isn't true.
- Avoid complex jargon. Only one of the panel is medically qualified.
- Avoid using expressions such as 'the patient admitted to' (e.g. suicidal thoughts) or 'the patient denied' (e.g. using illicit drugs). The words admitted and denied have pejorative implications. 'The patient said' has no such interpretation. We accept that repeatedly using this phrase doesn't make for interesting reading, but this isn't a novel!

- Avoid negative adjectives describing the patient. For example, don't describe patients as violent. Describe specific incidents of violence. The former may cause offence (because the patient believes their violence to have been justified), the latter doesn't.

- If the patient has a different view, include their version in the report. For example, 'The patient punched the nurse on the back of the head. The patient says he did this because he heard the nurse call him "a ..." [something offensive – use the patient's words]. Staff believe this was an auditory hallucination.' Patients really appreciate having their point of view reported.

- One of the most common areas of disagreement is whether or not the patient will continue to take medication after discharge. The patient will nearly always confirm that they will adhere fully. Saying that you don't believe the patient will probably cause arguments with the patient and solicitor and may lead the Tribunal to ask if you ever trust patients. Far better to describe what has happened in relation to adherence on previous occasions and, if appropriate, during the current admission. For example, 'I cannot say whether or not the patient will continue to take the prescribed medication. What I note is that on the last three occasions the patient stopped his medication within 2 weeks of discharge and was found to be trying to avoid taking it during this admission as recently as a week ago.' A similar example is when the patient states they will stay off illicit drugs. Restrict yourself to describing the patient's known use or refusal to comply with testing. Only give an opinion about the patient's future behaviour if specifically asked to do so by members of the Tribunal or the patient's solicitor.

- It's easy to become frustrated with the patient's solicitor. Why are they trying to get the patient discharged when it's so obvious the patient needs to be in hospital? It's important to remember that, although our job, and that of the Approved Mental Health Professional and Tribunal, is to do what's best for the patient and society, that isn't the solicitor's role. Their role is to try to achieve what the patient wants. They may say things that you think are ridiculous. Sometimes they say things that are so bizarre that they will distance themselves by using an expression such as 'I am instructed to say ...'. Everyone is doing their job to the best of their ability.

- Always say something – as much as possible – positive about the patient.

- Accept that, although in your (and hopefully the team's) opinion you are recommending the most appropriate medical care for your patient, if the Tribunal does not agree with you, it is not saying that you're wrong. It is just saying that your recommendations for management mustn't be forced on the patient. For example, a patient with paranoid schizophrenia regularly used illicit drugs (Mr M, whom we mentioned in Chapter 8). He was compliant with his depot medication, in that he didn't refuse it, but he often forgot his appointments. The Tribunal declined to discharge him because of the risk of relapse owing to his chaotic lifestyle. He appealed to the Upper Tribunal, which allowed his appeal on the grounds that his use of illicit drugs couldn't be relied on to justify detention where the evidence didn't show a link between the drug-taking and a relapse of the mental disorder.[20]

Two additional personal but possibly more contentious views are as follows:

- Don't withhold information from the patient (i.e. don't submit a 'confidential' report). First, patients have the right to know the basis on which they are being detained. Without this knowledge they cannot know how to change their behaviour as required. Second, there is a good chance they will find out anyway and this will harm relationships.

- Don't ever represent the detaining authority. It is far easier and better to be a humble witness giving your medical opinion, rather than to be the person who is locking the patient up.

What Are the Options If You Believe the Tribunal Has Got It Seriously Wrong?

The Tribunal has discharged your patient from compulsion or detention.

If you believe the Tribunal made an error in law, or conducted the hearing in a way that was far removed from proper procedures (e.g. they refused to let you, the Responsible Clinician, speak), then the detaining authority can appeal to the Upper Tribunal. This would entail involving the detaining authority's solicitors and following their advice.

Alternatively, if you become aware of information that was unknown to the Tribunal at the hearing, and that is so significant that you truly believe it would have changed the decision made, you may consider recommending re-detaining the patient. Perhaps you have new serious information about the patient's risk history or the patient's condition markedly deteriorates after the hearing. The decision on whether or not to make a new application for detention will, of course, rest with the Approved Mental Health Professional (or Nearest Relative).

More difficult is what to do if the patient tells the Tribunal that they will continue taking medication, or will stay in hospital informally, but, on being discharged from detention by the Tribunal, immediately refuses medication or undertakes their own discharge from hospital. The former problem, stopping taking medication, was addressed by Lord Bingham: if the risk to the patient is substantially increased by stopping the medication, then this may be grounds for re-detention.[21] The latter problem hasn't yet been resolved. On the one hand, the patient's decision to undertake their own discharge from hospital is significant new information. On the other, the patient isn't truly discharged from detention if they must stay in hospital (or for that matter take medication) or they will be re-detained. It is Hobson's choice for a patient to be told 'Do as I say without compulsion or you'll do as I say with compulsion!'. Because it is unlawful for a Tribunal to discharge a patient to conditions that amount to deprivation of liberty, we just wonder whether it should be considered unlawful for a Tribunal to discharge a patient from detention on the condition that they remain in hospital informally, given that they would in fact be re-detained under the MHA if they tried to leave.

Finally, be reassured that even if the Tribunal hearing is organised quickly, and held soon after the patient is detained, and discharges the patient, this does not in any way suggest that the initial detention was wrong. Should the patient ask for a judicial review of the original decision, the test is the usual Bolam-type standard (see Chapter 3, 'The Bolam Test'). The judge in one case said: 'The question I have to ask is whether, faced with the information that is recorded in the contemporaneous documents, the two mental health professionals who made the decision that they did, were acting outside of the boundaries of what was reasonable for a clinician or two clinicians to have done at the time?'[22]

Chapter 10

Special Provisions in Relation to Minors

There is no minimum age for the detention of minors under the MHA. Whether to use the Children Act 1989 or the MHA depends on the purpose of the detention and, therefore, on the most appropriate place for the young person to be detained. If the primary reason for detention is because the young person is mentally disordered and needs medical treatment in hospital, then the MHA is appropriate. But if the main requirement is care and control because of disturbed behaviour, then secure accommodation under the Children Act may be the better choice.

Admission to Hospital for the Assessment or Treatment of Mental Disorder

- For capacitous 16- and 17-year-olds:
  - informal if consenting; or
  - MHA if refusing.

- For incapacitous 16- and 17-year-olds:
  - MCA unless the person needs to be deprived of their liberty (Deprivation of Liberty Safeguards do not apply to under-18s), in which case:
    - parental consent if within the 'scope of parental responsibility' (previously referred to as the 'zone of parental control') (England); or
    - MHA if outside the 'scope of parental responsibility' (England).

- For competent under-16s:
  - informal if consenting; or
  - parental consent if refusing and within the 'scope of parental responsibility' (England); or
  - MHA.

- For incompetent under-16s:
  - parental consent if within the 'zone of parental control' (England); or
  - MHA.

Notes

- The preceding information relates to admission to hospital. Unless detained under the MHA, there will need to be a reassessment of the young person's capacity/competence and consent in relation to medical treatment (because capacity and consent are decision-specific).
- Guardianship cannot be used for a person under the age of 16.
- If practicable, one of the MHA assessing team (the two Registered Medical Practitioners and the Approved Mental Health Professional (AMHP)) should be trained in child and adolescent mental health services (CAMHS). The MHA Code of Practice (England) states:

> At least one of the people involved in the assessment of a person who is under 18 years old, ie one of the two medical practitioners or the AMHP, should be a clinician specialising in CAMHS. Where this is not possible, a CAMHS clinician should be consulted as soon as possible. In cases where the child or young person has complex or multiple needs, other clinicians may need to be involved, eg a learning disability CAMHS consultant where the child or young person has a learning disability.

For Wales, see Appendix A1.9.

Suitable Accommodation

For young people, whether informal or detained, the MHA (section 131A) requires that:

(2) The managers of the hospital shall ensure that the patient's environment in the hospital is suitable having regard to his age (subject to his needs).

(3) For the purpose of deciding how to fulfil the duty ... the managers shall consult a person who appears to them to have knowledge or experience of cases involving patients who have not attained the age of 18 years which makes him suitable to be consulted.

The MHA Code of Practice (England) lists the following as generally necessary to fulfil these requirements:[1]

- appropriate physical facilities;
- staff with the right training, skills and knowledge to understand and address the specific needs of children and young people;
- a hospital routine that will allow young patients' personal, social and educational development to continue as normally as possible; and
- access to the same educational opportunities as their peers, in so far as that is consistent with their ability to make use of them, considering their mental state.

For Wales, see Appendix 1, section A1.10.

This does not mean that no one under the age of 18 may be admitted to an adult ward. For patients approaching 18 years of age with particular needs, an adult ward may be the most 'suitable' environment. Services are required to notify the Care Quality Commission when a child or young person under 18 years of age is placed in a psychiatric ward or unit intended for adults, where the placement lasts for a continuous period of longer than 48 hours.

Consent to Treatment

Consent to treatment of minors (children and young people aged under 18 years) is even more complex and, unless you are very familiar with law in this area, specialist advice should be sought.

Minors Aged 16 and 17

Since the Family Law Reform Act 1969, 16- and 17-year-olds have been able to consent to medical treatment. It was assumed for many years that this meant they could also refuse treatment. However, Lord Donaldson said that this wasn't so: they could consent, but not refuse.[2] This anomaly has now been corrected for 16- and 17-year-olds, who are largely in the same legal position as adults where consenting to, or refusing, medical treatment for mental disorder is concerned, i.e. consent is required if the patient has capacity and the MCA applies if capacity is lacking. There are two differences, in relation to consent to treatment, between young people of this age and people aged 18 and over.

First, they may be unable to make the required decision for reasons other than that they lack capacity. As the MHA Code of Practice for England states:

> When assessing a young person's capacity to make the decision in question, practitioners should be aware that in some cases a young person may be unable to make a decision for reasons other than an impairment of, or a disturbance in the functioning of, their mind or brain (even if that is only temporary). In such cases, the person will not lack capacity within the meaning of the MCA. For example, a young person who is informed that they need to be admitted into hospital may, in the particular circumstances of the case, be unable to make a decision. This might be because they find themselves in an unfamiliar and novel situation, having never before been asked to absorb that type and quantity of information, or they are worrying about the implications of deciding one way or the other.

Second, their capacitous refusal may be overridden by a court, discussed below. In one case, the judge declared that it was lawful for the hospital's doctors to treat a 17-year-old girl following a drug overdose despite her refusal to consent to the treatment.[3]

Minors under 16 Years of Age

The courts have decided that children under the age of 16 may have the competence to consent to a treatment, depending on maturity of the child and the complexity of the treatment. This is commonly referred to as Gillick competence, after one of the parties in a court case: 'the parental right to determine whether or not their minor child below the age of sixteen will have medical treatment terminates if and when the child achieves a sufficient understanding and intelligence to enable him or her to understand fully what is proposed'.[4] It's worth noting that this test is rather stricter than that for adults!

Now this is where it gets more difficult. For this group, unlike 16- and 17-year-olds, the parental right to control a minor may extend beyond where the minor does not have the competence to determine what treatment is appropriate for their benefit and protection. 'A right of determination is wider than a right of consent .... In a case in which the "Gillick competent" child refuses treatment, but the parents consent, that consent enables treatment to be undertaken lawfully.'[5] On the other hand, it is suggested that the Human Rights Act, which this case preceded, may have changed things. In a case in which a mother challenged the Department of Health's advice in relation to the right of health professionals to keep medical advice to a minor confidential, the judge said: 'As a matter of principle, it is difficult to see why a parent should still retain an Article 8 [of the European Convention on Human Rights] right to parental authority relating to a medical decision where the young person concerned understands the advice provided by the medical professional and its implications.'[6] The MHA Code of Practice (England) advises that, if a capacitous young person refuses consent to treatment, it is not wise to rely on the consent of a person with parental responsibility. (For Wales, see Appendix 1, section A1.7.) The MHA Code of Practice for England states:

> Parental consent should not be relied upon when the child is competent or the young person has capacity to make the particular decision. The effect of section 131(4) of the Act in relation to the informal admission to hospital of a 16 or 17 year old, who has capacity, is that parental consent cannot be relied upon to override that young person's decision about their admission. In relation to decisions about such a young person's treatment, it is inadvisable to rely on the consent of a person with parental responsibility to treat a young person who has capacity to make the decision and has refused the treatment. Similarly, in relation to children, it is not advisable to rely on the consent of a parent with parental responsibility to admit or treat a child who is competent to make the decision and does not consent to it. Although in the past the courts have found that a person with parental responsibility can overrule their child's refusal, such decisions were made before the introduction of the HRA and since then court decisions concerning children and young people have given greater weight to their views.

The judgment in the recent case of *X (A Child)*[7] sets out the case law around consent to or refusal of treatment by those:

- under the age of 16 who are not Gillick competent;
- who are under the age of 16, but declared to be Gillick competent; and
- aged 16 and 17 when questions of competence are replaced by those of mental capacity.

The decision was that the court, in the exercise of its inherent jurisdiction, will have the right to overrule the child's (i.e. someone who has not reached the age of 18) decision, 'either, as the case may be, vetoing some procedure to which the child has consented or directing that the child should undergo some procedure to which the child is objecting'. Despite the judicial clarification, this is still a very difficult area. Other than in an emergency, legal advice, on a case-by-case basis, may be required. However, it does appear unlikely that doctors will proceed using the legal authority of the parents of competent or capacitous children.

If the child or young person lacks competence (under-16s) or capacity (16 and over) to consent, then parents, guardians or the courts can consent on their behalf. But the MHA Code of Practice for England states that two key questions must be asked. First: 'Is this a decision that a parent should reasonably be expected to make?' Factors to take into consideration include: the type and invasiveness of the intervention; the age, maturity and understanding of the young person; the extent to which the decision accords with the wishes of the young person; whether or not the young person tries to 'resist the decision'; and, if they previously had competence/capacity, whether or not they expressed a view on the proposed intervention. Second: 'Are there any factors that might undermine the validity of parental consent?' The Code advises that the parents' ability to make the relevant decision or act in their child's best interests are important considerations, as is whether there is agreement or conflict between the parents.

The parents of a 15-year-old suffering from attention deficit hyperactivity disorder, Asperger syndrome and Tourette syndrome, who was not Gillick competent in relation to his residence or care arrangement, wished to authorise his deprivation of liberty in a residential unit following his discharge from hospital. The judge said:

> I am satisfied that the circumstances in which D is accommodated would amount to a deprivation of liberty but for his parents' consent to his placement there. I am satisfied that, on the particular facts of this case, the consent of D's parents to his placement at Hospital B, with all of the restrictions placed upon his life there, falls within the 'zone of parental responsibility'. In the exercise of their parental responsibility for D, I am satisfied they have and are able to consent to his placement.[8]

It then fell to the Supreme Court to decide whether it is within the scope (note the change of word) of parental responsibility to consent to living arrangements for a 16- or 17-year-old child (who lacks relevant decision-making capacity) which amount to a deprivation of liberty.[9] The Supreme Court, by a narrow majority, concluded it is not. Lady Hale observed while both the child's parents and the local authority had his best interests at heart, 'this will not always be the case'. Therefore, a public authority seeking to impose measures which satisfy the 'acid test' in relation to a 16- or 17-year-old who lacks capacity must seek legal authorisation beyond parental consent, i.e. a court order or Liberty Protection Safeguards (when in force). For the time being at least, outside of the MHA, a court order is not required for under-16s where parental consent is obtained.

One final point: termination of pregnancy, sterilisation and withdrawal of treatment for severely disabled minors all require a court order.

Electroconvulsive Therapy

Both detained and informal under-18s can only be given ECT (except in an emergency):
- if they are capacitous/competent – with their consent and a SOAD certificate;
- if they lack capacity/competence:
  . if informal (and not against the decision of a court or court deputy) – with the consent of a parent or guardian and a SOAD certificate;
  . if detained – with a SOAD certificate.

Referrals to the Tribunal

The Hospital Managers must refer the patient to the Tribunal annually, unless the patient has already appealed.

How to Become Section 12 Approved and/or an Approved Clinician

In England, section 12 (strictly speaking, section 12(2)) and Approved Clinician approval are granted by section 12 and Approved Clinician panels on behalf of the Secretary of State. The qualifying requirements, which we summarise here, are set out in the Secretary of State for Health's instructions.[1] Please refer to that document for the complete list.

> **Note**
>
> If in doubt as to whether or not you meet the required criteria to become a section-12-approved doctor or an Approved Clinician, you should seek advice from your local approval panel.

Only Registered Medical Practitioners with a licence to practise may be section 12 and Approved Clinician approved. Registered Medical Practitioners who are Approved Clinicians are automatically section 12 approved. England and Wales give mutual recognition to section 12 approval. There are provisions to enable psychiatrists, general practitioners and forensic medical examiners to become section 12 approved. There are no specific statutory requirements other than that the doctor must have 'special experience in the diagnosis or treatment of mental disorder'. We have no idea why 'or' rather than 'and'!

> **Note**
>
> Registered Medical Practitioners who are Approved Clinicians are automatically section 12 approved and remain section 12 approved while they continue to be Approved Clinicians. This seems to cause confusion.

Approved Clinicians must have statutory competencies. Proof of attainment of the required competencies is established by portfolio for all professionals other than Registered Medical Practitioners who are on the General Medical Council's Specialist Register for psychiatry. For them, being on the Specialist Register is accepted as proof of competencies. The requirements for Registered Medical Practitioners who are not on the Specialist Register are the same as for the other qualifying professional groups. Approved Clinicians who wish to be approved in both England and Wales need to apply through the appropriate channels in each jurisdiction. Unlike section 12 approval, Approved Clinician approval is not mutually recognised.

There are a number of requirements, in addition to the professional ones, and these are listed below. You will note that both approvals require attendance at an approved 2-day course. For reasons that are beyond us, some colleagues seem to think that the requirement is simply to pay for a 2-day course and attend only part of it. This is incorrect. Attendance throughout the 2 days is required. There are special provisions to enable higher psychiatric trainees to take up locum consultant posts that include Approved Clinician status.

Note

For specialists who qualified outside England and Wales, the national guidelines for section 12 state that the doctor has to hold a substantive post with a minimum of 3 months of psychiatric practice in England or Wales.

The period of approval can be between 1 and 5 years. Doctors in substantive posts will usually be approved for 5 years, but may be approved for a shorter period. Applicants will be given reasons if this is the case.

For guidance for Wales, see Appendix 1.

Who Can Be Section 12 Approved?

Section 12 approval is open to any Registered Medical Practitioner with a licence to practise who has special experience in the diagnosis or treatment of mental disorder and fulfils one of the following five requirements:

(1) is a Member or Fellow of the Royal College of Psychiatrists; or

(2) is a Member of the Royal College of General Practitioners and has 3 years' experience in a salaried or principal permanent post with substantial experience in the diagnosis or treatment of mental disorder; 4 months or more of this experience must have been in a supervised psychiatric training post approved by the Royal College of Psychiatrists or the Royal College of General Practitioners;

or

(3) has 4 years' experience:

- in a psychiatric training post or a non-consultant career grade post (which includes training or supervision equivalent to that recognised by the Royal College of Psychiatrists) or a permanent salaried or principal psychiatrist post with substantial experience in the diagnosis and treatment of mental disorder;

or

- as general practitioner on the performers' list, with at least 4 months in a supervised, approved (by the Royal College of Psychiatrists or Royal College of General Practitioners) psychiatric training post;

and

- provides evidence of two competently undertaken MHA assessments supervised by a section 12 doctor who is also either a Member of the Royal College of Psychiatrists or on the Specialist Register as a specialist in psychiatry;

or

(4) is on the Specialist Register in psychiatry and has a minimum of 3 months' psychiatric practice in England or Wales and provides evidence of two competently undertaken MHA assessments supervised by a section 12 doctor;

or

(5) is a Member of the Faculty of Forensic and Legal Medicine of the Royal College of Physicians with evidence of:

- at least 4 years' post-registration clinical experience in areas relevant to the assessment of mental disorder, at least 4 months of which must be in a supervised psychiatric training post;

and

- at least 6 months' full-time or 12 months' part-time employment as a forensic physician;

and

- two competently undertaken MHA assessments supervised by a section 12 doctor.

What Else Is Required?

- an enhanced criminal record certificate;
- completion of a section 12 induction training course within 12 months of the application for approval, or a renewal course if already section 12 approved;
- evidence of satisfactory continuing professional development;
- an up-to-date curriculum vitae (CV) and two references; one of the referees must have worked with you; one must be a section-12-approved consultant psychiatrist, and the other must be an Approved Clinician, or a section-12-approved consultant psychiatrist, or the person responsible for your professional appraisal, or an Approved Mental Health Professional who works with you, or your current medical or clinical director.
- evidence of continuing involvement in the diagnosis or treatment of mental disorder within the preceding 12 months, for example:
  . employment in a clinical post;
  . acting as a Responsible Clinician or Approved Clinician;
  . acting as a Medical Member of a Mental Health Tribunal;
  . acting as a Second Opinion Appointed Doctor;
  . presentation of oral or written evidence to courts in relation to Part III of the MHA, the MCA or the Children Act.
  . completion of two or more MHA assessments.

Who Can Be an Approved Clinician?

- Registered Medical Practitioners with a licence to practise;
- first-level nurses whose field of practice is mental health or learning disability;
- registered occupational therapists;
- chartered psychologists; and
- registered social workers.

What Else Is Required?

- The relevant competencies, as outlined in the next section.
- An Enhanced Criminal Record Certificate.
- Completion of an Approved Clinician induction training course within 2 years of the application for approval, or a renewal course if already an Approved Clinician.
- Evidence of satisfactory continuing professional development.
- An up-to-date CV and two references. One of the referees must have worked with you and one (it might be the same one) must be your current or most recent medical or clinical director (if you're on a training programme recognised by the Royal College of Psychiatrists, the referee may be the programme director or equivalent); one must be an Approved Clinician and the other must be one of the following: an Approved Clinician; a section-12-approved consultant psychiatrist; or an Approved Mental Health Professional with whom you have worked in the past 12 months.

Competencies for Approved Clinicians

The following excerpt is from the rules for being appointed as an Approved Clinician.[2]

Relevant competencies for approved clinicians

1. A person must have the skills and competencies set out in paragraphs 2 to 9 below.

The role of the approved clinician and responsible clinician

2. A comprehensive understanding of the role, legal responsibilities and key functions of the approved clinician and the responsible clinician.

Legal and policy framework

3. (1) Applied knowledge of—

    (a) mental health legislation, related codes of practice and national and local policy and guidance;

    (b) other relevant legislation, codes of practice and national and local policy guidance, in particular, relevant parts of the Human Rights Act 1998, the Mental Capacity Act 2005, the Children Act 1989 and the Children Act 2004; and

    (c) relevant guidance issued by the National Institute for Health and Clinical Excellence (NICE).

   (2) In the above paragraph 'relevant' means relevant to the decisions likely to be taken by an approved clinician or responsible clinician.

Assessment

4. (1) Ability to—

    (a) identify the presence of mental disorder;

    (b) identify the severity of the disorder; and

    (c) determine whether the disorder is of a kind or degree warranting compulsory detention.

(2) Ability to assess all levels of clinical risk, including risks to the safety of the patient and others within an evidence-based framework for risk assessment and management.

(3) Ability to undertake mental health assessments incorporating biological, psychological, cultural and social perspectives.

Treatment

5. (1) Understanding of—

   (a) mental health related treatments, which include physical, psychological and social interventions;
   (b) different evidence based treatment approaches and their applicability to different patients; and
   (c) the range of appropriate treatments and treatment settings which can be provided in the least restrictive environment and will deliver the necessary health and social outcomes.

   (2) High level of skill in determining whether a patient has capacity to consent to treatment.
   (3) Ability to formulate, review appropriately and lead on treatment in relation to which the clinician is appropriately qualified in the context of a multi-disciplinary team.
   (4) Ability to communicate clearly the aims of the treatment to patients, carers and the team.

Care Planning

6. Ability to manage and develop care plans which combine health (including measures relating to physical and psychological health and medication), social services (including housing and employment) and other resources, preferably within the context of the Care Programme Approach.

Leadership and Multi-Disciplinary Team Working

7. (1) Ability to effectively lead a multi-disciplinary team.
   (2) Ability to assimilate the (potentially diverse) views and opinions of other professionals, patients and carers, whilst maintaining an independent view.
   (3) Ability to manage and take responsibility for making decisions in complex cases without the need to refer to supervision in each individual case.
   (4) Understanding and recognition of the limits of the person's own skills and an ability to seek professional views from others to inform a decision, for example through peer review and appraisal.

Equality and Cultural Diversity

8. (1) Up-to-date knowledge and understanding of relevant equality issues.
   (2) Ability to identify, challenge, and where possible and appropriate redress discrimination and inequality in relation to approved clinician practice.
   (3) Understanding of the need to sensitively and actively promote equality and diversity.
   (4) Understanding of how cultural factors and personal values can affect practitioners' judgements and decisions concerning the application of mental health legislation and policy.

Communication

9. (1) Ability to communicate effectively with professionals, patients, carers and others, particularly in relation to decisions taken and the underlying reasons for these.

   (2) Ability to keep appropriate records and an awareness of the legal requirements in relation to record keeping, including the processing of all personal data or sensitive personal data (as both terms are defined in the Data Protection Act 1998) in accordance with that Act.

   (3) Understanding of, and ability to manage, the competing requirements of confidentiality and effective information sharing, to the benefit of the patient and other stakeholders.

   (4) Ability to compile and complete statutory documentation and to provide written reports as required of an approved clinician.

   (5) Ability to present evidence to courts and tribunals.

Note

If you stop being on the relevant professional register for any reason (e.g. suspension), then you also stop being section 12 approved and/or an Approved Clinician.

Applying for Approval (England) for Section 12 and/or Approved Clinician Status

Although the panels' processes are similar (and more in line with each other than previously), they are not identical. Everyone applying for approval, either under section 12 or as an Approved Clinician, should check the process with their local panel. Some of the important points are listed below:

- You must be sure that you have the qualifications, experience and, to be an Approved Clinician, competencies required to meet the approval criteria and be able to produce the evidence required by your approval panel. Remember that you will need to provide referees (make sure you give up-to-date contact details), your CV, evidence of attendance at the relevant course, evidence of continuing professional development or further medical education, for trainee doctors your most recent Annual Review of Competence Progression outcome, and your criminal record check. Where required, you will also need to show that you have completed two supervised MHA assessments.

- Evidence of attainment of the required competencies to be an Approved Clinician is by portfolio unless you are a Registered Medical Practitioner on the General Medical Council's Specialist Register for psychiatry. Details of exactly what the portfolio should contain must be discussed with your approval panel. Approval of a portfolio may take many months.

- If you are a Registered Medical Practitioner in your final year of higher specialist training in psychiatry and wish to take up a locum consultant post, you need to provide a letter from your training programme director confirming that you are within 12 months of your expected Certificate of Completion of Training date,

making satisfactory progress in your training scheme and have been offered an acting-up consultant post for which you require Approved Clinician status.
- Approval always takes several weeks and may take much longer where references need to be checked. So, for example, CT3s requiring approval as section 12 doctors before starting ST4 posts are advised to contact their Section 12 Office about 3 months in advance.
- Attending a course does not confer approval.
- For Registered Medical Practitioners, being section 12 approved does not mean that you are an Approved Clinician (although being an Approved Clinician does mean you are section 12 approved).

Postscript

We must end with the following quote from Lord Justice Munby:[3]

> The fact is that all life involves risk, and the young, the elderly and the vulnerable are exposed to additional risks and to risks they are less well equipped than others to cope with. But just as wise parents resist the temptation to keep their children metaphorically wrapped up in cotton wool, so too we must avoid the temptation always to put the physical health and safety of the elderly and the vulnerable before everything else. Often it will be appropriate to do so, but not always. Physical health and safety can sometimes be bought at too high a price in happiness and emotional welfare. The emphasis must be on sensible risk appraisal, not striving to avoid all risk, whatever the price, but instead seeking a proper balance and being willing to tolerate manageable or acceptable risks as the price appropriately to be paid in order to achieve some other good – in particular to achieve the vital good of the elderly or vulnerable person's happiness. What good is it making someone safer if it merely makes them miserable?

It's an important message for those of us involved with the process of depriving people of their liberty and forcing treatment on those who don't want it.

Chapter 2

Reform of the Mental Health Act for England

In a wider legal milieu, it is typical for laws, including mental health legislation, to be reviewed and amended periodically as society progresses and services evolve. Prior to the June 2017 election, in an interview, Prime Minister Theresa May pledged to 'rip up the 1983 Act and introduce in its place a new law which finally confronts the discrimination and unnecessary detention that takes place too often'. She argued that the key reason for the increase in detentions is the 'discriminatory use of a law passed more than three decades ago'. Review of mental health law was then included in the government's legislative agenda in the Queen's speech of 21 June 2017.

The Wessely Review

In December 2018, an independent review of the MHA, chaired by Professor Sir Simon Wessely, completed its work and made recommendations for statutory reform of the MHA.[1]

The purpose of the review was to address the issues of:

- the rising rates of people being detained under the Act;
- the disproportionate number of people from black and minority ethnic groups detained under the Act;
- whether some processes relating to the Act are in line with a modern mental health system.

In response, a government White Paper[2] was published in January 2021. Accepting most of the recommendations, a number of changes for consultation were proposed.

Four principles, developed by the review, to shape the approach to reforming legislation, policy and practice are:

- choice and autonomy – ensuring service users' views and choices are respected;
- least restriction – ensuring the Act's powers are used in the least restrictive way;
- therapeutic benefit – ensuring patients are supported to get better, so they can be discharged from the Act;
- the person as an individual – ensuring patients are viewed and treated as individuals.

The government proposals for legislative change are (briefly):

- to tighten the criteria for detention under the MHA;
- to introduce more tribunal hearings to check on whether a patient's detention continues to be appropriate;
- to introduce Advance Choice Documents, which clinicians must take into account;

- to require that all detained patients must have a care and treatment plan;
- to introduce additional safeguards when certain forms of treatment are being provided without consent, e.g. electroconvulsive therapy in the face of a person's refusal;
- the Nominated Person (NP) to replace the Nearest Relative who the patient can personally select to represent them. The NP will have the same rights and powers as Nearest Relatives have now;
- to expand the role of Independent Mental Health Advocates;
- tightening criteria for use of Community Treatment Orders;
- in relation to the MHA/MCA interface, the intention is to await impact of the implementation of the Liberty Protection Safeguards;
- to improve the powers available to health professionals in A&E departments so that individuals in need of urgent mental healthcare receive it;
- to introduce a new power of 'supervised discharge', which would enable the discharge of a restricted patient with conditions amounting to a deprivation of that person's liberty;
- to revise section 3 criteria so that autism and learning disabilities are not considered to be mental disorders for this purpose.

The government has subsequently published its response to the consultation[3] and we wait to see how the legislative agenda and timescales evolve.

Appendix 1: Guidelines and Forms for Wales

A1.1 Additional Welsh Amendments to the Mental Health Act 1983

The Welsh Parliament, which superseded the Welsh Assembly in 2020, has the authority to pass Acts of the Welsh Parliament in relation to matters devolved from the UK Parliament. The main changes to the Mental Health Act 1983 (MHA) introduced in 2011 and 2012 are summarised below. This list is not exhaustive and full details may be found in the relevant statutes.

The Assembly has made a number of changes to the MHA for implementation in Wales which were introduced in 2011 and 2012. Here, we summarise the main ones. This list is not exhaustive and full details may be found in the relevant statute.

- There will be a duty to carry out a mental health assessment on defined primary and secondary care patients, including patients liable to be detained under the MHA, those subject to guardianship, CTO patients and individuals who are 'receiving secondary mental health services'.

The purpose of the assessment is to obtain:

an analysis of an individual's mental health which identifies—

(a) the local primary mental health treatment (if any) which might improve or prevent a deterioration in the individual's mental health (any treatment so identified must be provided: see sections 3 and 5); and

(b) other services (if any) which might improve or prevent a deterioration in the individual's mental health.

- There will be a statutory requirement to appoint a care coordinator, who has a number of defined responsibilities. Patients must have written care plans with defined outcomes that the plans are designed to achieve. Regulations may determine the form and content of care and treatment plans.

- The roles and responsibilities of Independent Mental Health Advocates are extended to include (section 130I):

- all patients 'liable to be detained under this Act (other than under section 135 or 136 below) and the hospital or registered establishment in which he is liable to be detained is situated in Wales';

- patients 'subject to guardianship under this Act and the area of the responsible local social services authority within the meaning of section 34(3) above is situated in Wales'; and

- 'a community patient and the responsible hospital is situated in Wales'. Informal patients are also included if (section 130J):

  (a) the patient is an in-patient at a hospital or registered establishment situated in Wales;

  (b) the patient is receiving treatment for, or assessment in relation to, mental disorder at the hospital or registered establishment; and

  (c) no application, order, direction or report renders the patient liable to be detained under this Act.

A1.2 Principles of the MHA Code of Practice

The revised *Mental Health Act 1983: Code of Practice for Wales* sets out a slightly different set of guiding principles from those in the English Code. The following excerpts are from Chapter 1 of the current Code:

Dignity and respect

1.3 Practitioners performing functions under the Act should respect the rights and dignity of patients and their families and carers, while also ensuring their safety and that of others.

1.4 Patients, families and carers should be respected, listened to and their views positively valued, recorded and taken into account when decisions are made.

1.5 Patients should be offered treatment and care in supportive environments that are safe for them, staff and the public. The physical and cultural environment should support practitioners to deliver therapies which focus on patient recovery, other positive clinical and personal outcomes and also promote the maintenance of patients' dignity to the fullest extent possible.

1.6 Issues of faith, spirituality, religion and belief may be central to a patient's cultural needs in general and these must be considered when decisions about their care and treatment are being made.

Least restrictive option and maximising independence

1.7 Services should be provided in line with the presumption of capacity, be the least restrictive option, serve a person's best interests and maximise independence.

1.8 Retaining independence and promoting the patient's recovery should be central to all interventions under the Act. The least restrictive options should always be considered and alternatives to avoid the use of compulsory powers should be explored before making an application for admission. Where it is possible to treat a patient safely and lawfully without detaining them under the Act, the patient should not be detained.

1.9 Where an application for detention under the Act is made, the patient should be informed, in the most appropriate manner, of the reasons for, and purpose of, the detention. This is in addition to providing the patient with information on their statutory rights.

1.10 In making decisions under the Act, adherence to other legislation and guidance may also be relevant, including that on safeguarding. Mental health professionals should not view mental health and learning disability guidance in isolation, and should ensure their practice takes account of wider legislation and guidance.

1.11 If the Act is used, detention should be used for the shortest time necessary in the least restrictive hospital setting available, and be delivered as close as reasonably possible to a location that the patient identifies they would like to be close to (e.g. their home or close to a family member or carer). If appropriate treatment cannot be delivered in the hospital setting closest to the location identified by the patient then the reasons for this should be recorded.

1.12 Restrictions that apply to all patients in a particular setting (blanket or global restrictions) should be avoided and should never be for the convenience of the provider. Any restrictions should be the minimum necessary to safely provide the care and treatment required and should be the least restrictive to the person's rights and freedom to act.

1.13 It is important that care and treatment planning should begin when the patient is admitted to hospital in order to focus on seeking early discharge and providing after-care, if necessary, at the earliest opportunity.

Fairness, equality and equity

1.14 People taking decisions under the Act must recognise and respect the diverse needs, values and circumstances of each patient, including their age, disability, gender reassignment, marriage and civil partnership, pregnancy and maternity, race, religion or belief, sex and sexual orientation and culture, or any combination of these. There must be no unlawful discrimination and reasonable adjustments must be made. Individuals' protected characteristics should be taken into account and good practice followed in all aspects of care and treatment planning and implementation.

1.15 Ensuring effective communication between practitioners, patients and others who are concerned with the care of the patient is central to fair and equitable practice. Everything practicable must be done to overcome any barriers to communication that may exist.

1.16 Welsh speakers must be given the option of assessment, treatment and provision of information in line with the Welsh Language Standards (No. 1) Regulations 2015. The commissioners and providers of services must act in accordance with the Welsh Language Measure (Wales) 2011.

1.17 If a patient's language is neither English nor Welsh, or the person has a sensory impairment or other disability which impedes communication, assessments and all communication with patients should be conducted using an appropriate interpreter, who will address issues of both language and cultural interpretation. All information provided to patients, families and carers should be in their first language whenever possible. Treatment should be provided in an individual's first language or using an interpreter whenever practicable. This includes the use of British Sign Language.

Empowerment and involvement

1.18 Where assessment under the Act is required, patients should be empowered to be as fully involved in the assessment process as possible. Mental health professionals undertaking assessments should give due regard to patients' present and past wishes, including any advance decisions.

1.19 All patients should be enabled and given the opportunity to participate in planning, developing and reviewing their own care and treatment. Families, carers and relevant others should be involved when practicable. Care and treatment planning should draw on and build on patients' strengths and should seek to enable patients to progress towards recovery and to re-establish or maximise independence as soon as is safely practicable. Whenever possible, care and treatment should encourage a sense of hope and aspiration. Patients should also be supported to manage, in accordance with their wishes, as many other aspects of their lives as possible.

1.20 Patients must, and their families and carers should normally, be informed of the support that an independent mental health advocate (IMHA) or an independent mental capacity advocate (IMCA), where relevant, can provide.

1.21 The patient's choices and views should be recorded. Where a decision in the care and treatment plan is contrary to the wishes of the patient or others, the reasons for this should be explained to them and fully documented. As far as is practicable, patients should be encouraged and supported to develop advance statements of wishes and feelings.

Keeping people safe

1.22 Patient well-being and safety should be at the heart of all decision-making under the Act. This should be consistent with ensuring the well-being and safety of others when needed.

1.23 Patients, their families and/or carers and other relevant individuals should, where appropriate, be actively involved in assessing the risks posed to the health and safety of the patient and others. Patients should, wherever practicable, be involved in creating and implementing a risk management plan.

1.24 Decision-making should be open and transparent, subject to the need to manage information which, if disclosed, could harm the patient and/ or the well-being and safety of others.

1.25 The planning of a patient's discharge should begin prior to discharge and be in line with the Code of Practice for Parts 2 and 3 of the Measure.

Effectiveness and efficiency

1.26 Anyone made subject to compulsion under the Act must be provided with appropriate assessment and/or treatment and care, the purpose of which should be: to establish the presence of; to alleviate; to minimise the harm caused by; or prevent a worsening of, their mental disorder, or any of its symptoms or manifestations.

1.27 Health, social care and other relevant agencies should work together to ensure patients are provided with a range of mental health services that are effective, accessible, responsive and of high quality.

1.28 Staff should have sufficient skills, information and knowledge about the Act to support all their patients. There should be clear mechanisms for accessing specialist support for those with additional needs.

1.29 All relevant organisations should work together to ensure, as far as practicable, the duration of detention is minimised and safe discharge from hospital is facilitated, with appropriate support, if required.

A1.3 Section 2 or Section 3?

From Chapter 14 of the *Mental Health Act 1983: Code of Practice for Wales*:

Use of section 2 or section 3 of the Act
14.20 In deciding whether a person should be detained in hospital under the Act, careful consideration must be given to which section, if any, would be the most appropriate, particularly bearing in mind the principle of least restriction. Professional judgement must be applied in making this decision.

Section 2 pointers:

- An assessment as an in-patient must be carried out in order to produce a treatment plan.
- A judgement is required on whether the patient will accept treatment on a voluntary/informal basis after admission.
- A judgement has to be made on whether a proposed treatment, which can only be administered to the patient under Part 4 of the Act, is likely to be effective.
- The condition of a patient who has already been assessed, and who has been previously admitted compulsorily under the Act, is judged to have changed since the previous admission and further assessment is required.
- The diagnosis and/or prognosis of a patient's condition is unclear.
- It has not been possible to undertake any other assessment in order to formulate a treatment plan.

Section 3 pointers:

- The patient is considered to need compulsory admission for the treatment of a mental disorder, which is already known to his or her clinical team, and has recently been assessed by that team.
- The patient is detained under section 2 and assessment indicates a need for compulsory treatment under the Act beyond the existing period of detention. In such circumstances an application for detention under section 3 should be made at the earliest opportunity and should not be delayed until the end of the existing period of detention.

A1.4 Nearest Relative's Objection and Section 2 or 3

From Chapter 14 of the *Mental Health Act 1983: Code of Practice for Wales*:

14.21 Decisions [as to section 2 or 3] should not be influenced by the possibility that: . . .

- a patient's nearest relative objects to admission under section 3.

A1.5 Conflicts of Interest

From Chapter 39 of the *Mental Health Act 1983: Code of Practice for Wales*:

Conflicts of interest

39.1 Conflicts of interest may arise which prevent an approved mental health professional (AMHP) from making the application for a patient's detention or guardianship, and a doctor from making a recommendation supporting the application.

Conflicts of interest regulations

39.2 The Mental Health (Conflicts of Interest) (Wales) Regulations 2008 (the Regulations) set out the circumstances in which there is a potential conflict of interest such that an AMHP cannot make an application mentioned in section 11(1) of the Act, or a registered medical practitioner cannot make a medical recommendation for the purposes of an application mentioned in section 12(1) for a person to be admitted under the Act.

39.3 The potential conflict of interest may arise for a number of reasons. Those reasons are the existence of a professional, financial, business or personal relationship between that person and another assessor, or between that person and either the patient or, where the application is to be made by the patient's nearest relative.

Financial conflict

39.4 The Regulations state that where the application is for the admission of the patient to a registered establishment (i.e. an independent hospital), neither of the medical recommendations may be given by a registered medical practitioner who is on the staff of that hospital or who receives or has an interest in the receipt of any payments made on account of the maintenance of the patient.

39.5 This is not the case for doctors who work in NHS hospitals. The Regulations state that where the application is for the admission of the patient to a hospital which is not a registered establishment, one (but not more than one) of the medical recommendations may be given by a registered medical practitioner who is on the staff of that hospital or who receives or has an interest in the receipt of any payments made on account of the maintenance of the patient.

39.6 There will be a conflict of interest for financial reasons if the assessor stands to make a financial gain, dependent upon whether or not the assessor decides to make an application or give a medical recommendation. However, any fee paid to a practitioner in respect of an examination of a patient pursuant to section 12 of the Act or the provision of any recommendation as a result of such examination, will not be a financial gain for the purposes of the Regulations.

Business conflict

39.7 When considering a patient, an assessor will have a potential conflict of interest if that assessor is closely involved in the same business venture as another assessor, the patient or the patient's nearest relative including being a partner, a director, other office-holder or major shareholder of that venture.

Where the patient's nearest relative is making an application, an assessor will have a potential conflict of interest if he or she is closely involved in the same business venture as the nearest relative including being a partner, director, other office holder or major shareholder of that venture.

Professional conflict

39.8 The Regulations state that, when considering a patient, an assessor will have a potential conflict of interest for professional reasons if:

- the assessor works under the direction of, or is employed by, one of the other assessors considering the patient
- the assessor is a member of a team organised to work together for clinical purposes on a routine basis of which the other two assessors are also members.

39.9 Where the patient's nearest relative is making an application, an assessor will have a potential conflict of interest if:

- the assessor works under the direction of, or is employed by, that patient's nearest relative
- the assessor employs the patient's nearest relative or the nearest relative works under his or her direction
- the assessor is a member of a team organised to work together for clinical purposes on a routine basis of which the nearest relative is also a member.

39.10 When considering a patient, an assessor will have a potential conflict of interest if:

- the assessor works under the direction of, or is employed by, the patient
- employs the patient or the patient works under his or her direction
- the assessor is a member of a team organised to work together for clinical purposes on a routine basis of which the patient is also a member.

Personal conflict

39.11 An assessor will have a potential conflict of interest in considering a patient, if he or she is related to another assessor, the patient or the patient's nearest relative (if the nearest relative is making the application), the assessor should withdraw from the application process.

39.12 The Regulations set out the nature of the personal relationships pertinent to a personal conflict. An assessor is considered to be in a personal relationship with another assessor, the patient or the patient's nearest relative if he or she is:

- related to them in the first degree (parent, sister, brother, son or daughter, including step relationships)
- related to them in the second degree (uncle, aunt, grandparent, grandchild, first cousin, niece, nephew, parent-in-law, grandparent-in-law, grandchild-in-law, sister- or brother-in-law, son- or daughter-in-law, including step relationships)
- related to them as a half-sister or half-brother
- their spouse, ex-spouse, civil partner or ex-civil partner
- living with them as though they were their spouse or civil partner.

39.13 References to step relationships and in-laws, above, include those arising from civil partnership as well as marriage.

Emergency provision

39.14 The Regulations do not prevent an AMHP making an application or a registered medical practitioner giving a medical recommendation if there would otherwise be delay involving serious risk to the health or safety of the patient or others.

Other potential conflicts

39.15 There may be circumstances not covered by the Regulations where the assessor feels there is (or could be seen to be) a potential conflict of interest.

Assessors should work on the principle that in any situation where they believe the objectivity or independence of their decision in the application process is (or could be seen to be) undermined, then they should not become involved or should withdraw. This could include a therapeutic or pastoral relationship between any of the assessors or the assessors and the patient.

39.16 The Regulations do not cover potential conflicts of interest relating to a community treatment order (CTO). The responsible clinician (RC), who is responsible for making the decision as to whether to place a patient on a CTO, or any decision to revoke a CTO, should not have any financial interest in the outcome of the decision and should not be a relative of the patient. RCs should not be regarded as having a financial interest in a hospital solely because they work there.

39.17 These Regulations do not cover potential conflicts of interest relating to renewal of detention or guardianship. However, the persons involved in making the decision as to whether to renew the detention (the RC and other professionals consulted by the RC) or the guardianship (the appropriate practitioner) should not have any financial interest in the outcome of the decision.

39.18 The Act requires an AMHP to take an independent decision about whether or not to make an application under the Act. If an AMHP believes they are being placed under undue pressure to make, or not make, an application, they should raise this through the appropriate local channels. Local arrangements should be in place to deal with such situations.

A1.6 Factors to Consider in Deciding Whether or Not to Recommend a CTO

From Chapter 29 of the *Mental Health Act 1983: Code of Practice for Wales*:

29.10 CTOs should only be used when there is reasonable evidence to suggest there will be benefits to the patient. Such evidence may include:

- a clear link between non-concordance with medication and relapse which is likely to require treatment in hospital
- clear evidence there is a positive response to medication
- evidence the CTO will promote recovery
- evidence recall may be necessary (rather than informal admission or reassessment under the Act).

29.11 Other relevant factors will vary, but are likely to include the patient's current mental state, the patient's insight and attitude to treatment, and the circumstances into which the patient would be discharged.

29.12 Taken together, all these factors should help the responsible clinician to assess the risk of the patient's condition deteriorating after discharge, and inform the decision as to whether continued detention; a CTO or discharge from detention would be the right option for the patient at that particular time.

A1.7 Parental Consent

From Chapter 19 of the *Mental Health Act 1983: Code of Practice for Wales*:

19.25 Those with parental responsibility have a central role in relation to decisions about the admission and treatment of their child and parental responsibility should be established in line with the relevant circumstances of the child and associated legislation.

19.26 However parental consent should not be relied upon when a child under 16 is competent or the young person aged 16 and 17 has capacity to make the particular decision. Parental consent cannot be relied upon to override a young person aged 16 or 17's decision about their admission. Similarly, in relation to children under 16, it is not advisable to rely on the consent of a parent with parental responsibility to admit or treat a child who is competent to make the decision and does not consent to it.

A1.8 The Welsh Tribunal

Many of the rules relating to the Tribunal in Wales are quite different from the rules in England. The following excerpts are from *The Mental Health Review Tribunal for Wales Rules 2008.*[2]

Withholding documents or information likely to cause harm

17(1) The Tribunal must give a direction prohibiting the disclosure of a document or information to a person if it is satisfied that—

 (a) such disclosure would be likely to cause that person or some other person serious harm; and

 (b) having regard to the interests of justice that it is proportionate to give such a direction.

Request to appear at and take part in a hearing

26 The Tribunal may give a direction permitting or requesting any person to—

 (a) attend and take part in a hearing to such extent as the Tribunal considers appropriate; or

 (b) make written submissions in relation to a particular issue.

Use of the Welsh Language in the Welsh Tribunal

From *Practice Direction: First-Tier and Upper Tribunal. Use of The Welsh Language in Tribunals in Wales:*[3]

> If a Tribunal is deemed to be a Welsh Tribunal (usually because all the relevant people are resident in Wales) 'the Welsh language may be used by any party or witnesses or in any document placed before the Tribunal or [subject to certain conditions] at any hearing'.

From Chapter 1 of the *Mental Health Act 1983: Code of Practice for Wales*:

1.18 Welsh speakers should, where reasonably practicable or appropriate in the circumstances, be given the option of assessment, treatment and provision of information through the medium of Welsh. Service providers, who have Welsh language schemes, must act in accordance with their schemes.

A1.9 Professional Staff and the Detention of Minors

From Chapter 33 of the *Mental Health Act 1983: Code of Practice for Wales*:

33.11 If possible, all staff involved in the care and treatment of children should be child specialists. They must always have been vetted satisfactorily with the Criminal Records Bureau. If it is not possible to have such a specialist in charge of the child's treatment, arrangements should be made for the clinical staff caring for the child to have access to a practitioner who is a specialist in child and adolescent mental healthcare (CAMHS) – that is an experienced specialist practitioner who has been trained and practices in delivering the functions of tiers 2, 3 and/or 4 in the CAMHS Strategic Framework for Wales.

A1.10 Age-Appropriate Wards

From Chapter 33 of the *Mental Health Act 1983: Code of Practice for Wales*:

33.9 Children admitted to hospital for treatment of mental disorder should, subject to their needs, be accommodated suitably for their age. This means they should have appropriate physical facilities, staff with the right training to understand and address their specific needs as children, and a hospital routine that will allow their personal, social and educational development to continue as normally as possible.

A1.11 Section 12 Approval

Betsi Cadwaladr University Health Board is responsible for initial approval, re-approval, suspension and termination of Approved Clinicians and section 12(2) doctors in Wales. Clinicians making an application for approval should be aware that the guidance for both section 12 and Approved Clinician status can change.

From the Mental Health Act 1983 Section 12(2): Approval/Re-Approval Process and Criteria for Wales:[4]

7.4 Every Panel will comprise of two registered medical practitioners who are section 12 approved.

7.5 The Approval Panel will review the evidence provided. The Panel members will review the evidence independently of each other.

7.6 The Panel will make a recommendation to Betsi Cadwaladr University Health Board as to approval, re-approval or ending of approval. The Panel decision making process will be as follows:

  i. If both Panel Members are satisfied with the evidence received, the final recommendation will be submitted to the Approval Team for approval and ratification by the Board.

  ii. If the decision is not unanimous, the decision will be brought to the attention of the Approval Team. Further information may be requested.

  iii. If the Approving Panel does not consider that the candidate has met the requirements for approval; their reasoning will be given, together with advice as to what the applicant will need to do to fulfil the criteria.

  iv. The Board will receive a report detailing approval, re-approval and termination of approval at bimonthly Board meeting.

  v. The approval process will take a maximum of 7 weeks unless additional information is required from the applicant or their employer/referees. vi. Based on the recommendation of the Panel, the delegated officer of the Board will send a letter to the applicant informing them of the outcome.

7.7 Applicants must meet the following approval criteria before approval/re-approval will be given:-

All doctors will be required to submit an application form and evidence to an Approval Panel for initial approval and re-approval to ensure they meet the professional requirements to undertake Section 12 functions. In addition, the panel will require two references. Both referees must have worked with the applicant for a minimum of three months in the previous twelve months in England or Wales. Referees must be able to comment on the applicant's understanding of and ability to implement the Mental Health Act (1983). The All Wales AC and Section 12 Approvals Panel has reference template forms which applicants must send to their referees for completion. One of the referees must be a Consultant Psychiatrist who is a Section 12 Approved Doctor and the other referee must be either a second Section 12 Approved Doctor or Approved Mental Health Professional who have professional knowledge of the individual and their work for at least three months during the past twelve months and can confirm that they are able to carry out the duties of a Doctor approved under Section 12(2) of the Mental Health Act 1983. These references should be submitted by the individual together with the application form and evidence as follows:

i.   Satisfy the GMC Standards of Fitness to Practise (appendix 1).

ii. With effect from the 16th November 2009, all doctors will be required to be licensed medical practitioners to be approved under section 12(2) of the Mental Health Act 1983.

iii. Attend an approved section 12 induction training course within two years prior to making the application for initial approval. Attend an approved section 12 refresher course within the final two years of approval for re-approval.

iv. For GPs – have an up to date annual appraisal which evidences a satisfactory outcome in line with current GMC requirements.

For Psychiatrists – either be registered with the Royal College of Psychiatrists and provide a certificate of good standing for CPD purposes. Or, provide a satisfactory CPD log which has been signed by two members of the peer group. The CPD log must satisfy the Royal College of Psychiatrists criteria using the All Wales CPD form. Psychiatry Trainees to provide evidence of a satisfactory ARCP outcome.

v.   Provide an up to date curriculum vitae that provides evidence/practice examples of relevant experience to support application.

vi. Applicants for approval must satisfy at least one of the following sets of additional criteria from A or B. Applicants for re-approval must satisfy the criteria from C.

vii. A copy of the most recent Disclosure and Barring Scheme (DBS) certificate is required from Applicants who work through a Locum Employment Agency or who are independent practitioners. The DBS certificate must include checks against the DBS children's Barred List information and the DBS Adults' Barred List information.

Criteria A (New Applications)

1. Be a member or fellow of the Royal College of Psychiatrists, or the Royal College of General Practitioners, or be included on the Specialist Register of the GMC as a Specialist in Psychiatry (or equivalent speciality), or hold a GMC licence to practice as a Consultant Psychiatrist, or hold a post in the National Health Service as a Consultant Psychiatrist under the NHS International Fellowship Programme. New applicants for approval would normally be expected to have one of the above but would be considered without this depending on prior experience. and

2. Have three year equivalent whole time experience in Psychiatry or Primary Care as a GP principal/salaried practitioner, which is not a temporary post, and who is on the Medical Performers List, where there was special experience in the diagnosis or treatment of mental disorder either in the UK or in line with GMC Guidance as an Overseas Qualified Doctor. At least four months of experience must be in an approved supervised psychiatric training post and accredited training department or satisfy the criteria for GPwSI. An overseas

qualified doctor must first demonstrate their suitability for supervised practice under limited registration. After a period of limited registration those doctors may then apply for full registration on the basis that they have demonstrated their capability for unrestricted practice.

Criteria B

1. Have four years' equivalent whole time experience in Psychiatry or Primary Care as a GP Principal/salaried practitioner, which is not a temporary post, and who is on the Medical Performers List, where there was special experience in the diagnosis or treatment of mental disorder either in the UK or in line with GMC Guidance as an Overseas Qualified Doctor. At least four months of experience must be in an approved supervised psychiatric training post and accredited training department or satisfy the criteria for GPwSI. An overseas qualified doctor must first demonstrate their suitability for supervised practice under limited registration. After a period of limited registration those doctors may then apply for full registration on the basis that they have demonstrated their capability for unrestricted practice. and

2. Attend two supervised Mental Health Act assessments, within one year alongside a section 12 approved Doctor and achieve continuous satisfactory reports.

   Forensic Physicians, who are not Psychiatrists or General Practitioners on the Medical Performers List, must apply under Criteria B. They should be a member of the Faculty of Forensic and Legal Medicine of the Royal College of Physicians, have a reference from the local lead forensic physician which includes evidence with respect to training, and have experience which includes:-

(a) at least four years of clinical experience after registration as a member of the Faculty in areas considered by the approving body to be relevant to the assessment of mental disorder, whether gained in consecutive years or not, at least four months of which are in a supervised psychiatric training post;

(b) a minimum of six months' full time or twelve months' part time employment as a forensic physician, whether gained in consecutive years or not.

Criteria C (Applications for Re-approval)

1. Applications for re-approval are required to be submitted 7 weeks prior to current approval expiring. All doctors will be required to submit an application form and evidence to an approval panel to ensure they continue to meet the professional requirements to undertake section 12(2) functions. This includes General Practitioners who have previously been but are not currently on the Medical Performers List; and have previously been a section 12 doctor and the date of the end of the practitioner's latest period of approval as a section 12 doctor is within the twelve month period immediately preceding the date of the practitioner's application for a re-approval. and

2. Each doctor seeking re-approval will be required to undertake refresher training within the final two years of the current approval period.

All individuals must provide written confirmation (patient identifiable information removed) of one or more of the following:-

i. Undertaking at least two assessments under Part II of the Mental Health Act 1983 within the previous two years.

ii. Confirmation of active involvement as a medical member of the Mental Health

Review Tribunal for Wales or the First Tier Tribunal (HESC Chamber).

iii. Active involvement as a Second Opinion Appointed Doctor (SOAD) under the Mental Health Act 1983.

iv. Preparation of independent expert reports for Courts under Part 3 or the MHA, Mental Capacity Act, Deprivation of Liberty Safeguards or relevant legislation relating to children.

v. Undertaking assessments as a Second Opinion Appointed Doctor for the Care Quality Commission or the Healthcare Inspectorate Wales.

vi. Confirmation of having acted as a Responsible Clinician or a Section 12 Doctor in charge of the treatment of a patient.

vii. Attend two Mental Health Act assessments supervised by a Section 12 approved Doctor and achieve continuous satisfactory reports.

A1.12 Competencies to Be an Approved Clinician

From Schedule 2 of the *National Health Service (Wales) Act 2006: Mental Health Act 1983 Approved Clinician (Wales) Directions 2008:*[5]

1. **The role of the approved clinician:**

   1.1. A comprehensive understanding of the role, legal responsibilities and key functions of the approved clinician and the responsible clinician.

2. **Values based practice**

   2.1. The ability to identify and apply the range of appropriate and effective health and social care treatments and treatment settings which can be provided in the least restrictive methods for those dealt with or who may be dealt with under the 1983 Act.

   2.2. An understanding and respect of individuals' unique personal characteristics.

   2.3. Sensitivity to individuals' needs in terms of respect to the patient and the patient's choice, dignity and privacy whilst exercising the role of approved clinician or responsible clinician.

   2.4. The ability to promote the rights, dignity and self determination of patients consistent with their own needs and wishes, to enable them to contribute to the decisions made affecting their quality of life and liberty.

3. **Assessment:**

   3.1. The ability to identify the presence or absence of mental disorder and the severity of the disorder, including whether it is of a kind or degree warranting the use of detention under the 1983 Act.

   3.2. The ability to undertake a mental health assessment incorporating biological, psychological, cultural and social perspectives.

   3.3. The ability to assess all levels of clinical risk, and the safety of the patient and others within an evidence based framework for risk assessment and management.

   3.4. The ability to demonstrate a high level of skill in determining whether a patient has capacity to consent to treatment.

4. **Care Planning**

   4.1. Possession of the skills and knowledge necessary to undertake safe, effective and efficient care planning, including (but not limited to) being able to:

      (a) involve patients and (where appropriate) their families and carers in care planning;

      (b) assess patients' needs;

      (c) formulate individual care plans to meet identified needs;

(d) ensure that care plans are implemented as agreed;

(e) review and evaluate care plans (and revise as necessary).

5. Treatment

5.1. The skills and knowledge necessary to harness the specialist treatment expertise of the multidisciplinary team, for the benefit of the patient. To include (but not be limited to) an understanding of the roles and specialist competences of the various members of a multidisciplinary team, in relation to specific treatments and therapies.

5.2. Broad understanding of all mental health related treatments, i.e. physical, psychological and social interventions.

6. Leadership and Multi Disciplinary Team Working:

6.1. Possession of the skills and knowledge necessary to:

(a) lead effectively a multi-disciplinary team in the delivery of co-ordinated programmes of care, in order to meet the needs of patients for whom he or she is responsible;

(b) take into account the views and opinions of patients and (where appropriate) their families and carers when developing programmes of care involving the team;

(c) consider objectively the professional opinions of other colleagues within the team when formulating programmes of care, so as to ensure that care and treatment decisions are multi-disciplinary and based on sound evidence.

6.2. An advanced level of skills in making and taking responsibility for complex judgements and decisions, without referring to supervision in each individual case.

7. Equality and Cultural Diversity:

7.1. Demonstrates an up to date knowledge of race equality legislation and other equality issues, including disability, sexual orientation and gender.

7.2. Has a broad grasp of issues of social exclusion.

7.3. Understands the need to promote equality and diversity.

7.4. Aware of how cultural factors and personal values can affect practitioners' judgements and decisions in the application of mental health legislation.

7.5. Ability to identify, challenge, and where possible redress discrimination and inequality in all its forms in relation to approved clinician practice.

8. Mental Health Legislation and Policy:

8.1. Up to date working knowledge of:

(a) the Act;

(b) relevant NICE Guidelines:

(c) relevant parts of other related legislation (including the Mental Capacity Act 2005, the Human Rights Act 1998 and the Children Acts);

(d) all other relevant codes, national policies and protocols related to mental health;

(e) Case law relevant to the practice of approved clinicians and responsible clinicians.

9. Communication:

9.1. Able to communicate effectively with professions, service users, carers and others, particularly in relation to decisions taken and the underlying reasons for these.

9.2. Consideration of the needs of individuals for whom Welsh is their language of choice.

9.3. Able to demonstrate appropriate record keeping and an awareness of the legal requirements with respect to record keeping.

9.4. Ability to compile and complete statutory documentation and to provide written reports as required of an approved clinician.

5. Ability with regard to effective report writing.

6. Ability to competently present evidence both verbal and written, to courts and tribunals.

Notes

- Full guidance for approval as an Approved Clinician in Wales appears in *Mental Health Act 1983: Approval of Approved Clinicians (Wales).*[6]
- The applicant must have attended the Approved Clinician approval course not more than 2 years prior to being granted AC approval.
- Approved Clinicians who are Registered Medical Practitioners are automatically deemed to be section 12 approved.

A1.13 Care Coordination and Treatment Planning

The Explanatory Note to *Mental Health (Care Co-ordination and Care and Treatment Planning) (Wales) Regulations 2011:*[7]

Explanatory Note

1. These Regulations contain provisions about care co-ordination and care and treatment planning for patients using secondary mental health services (within the meaning of The Mental Health (Wales) Measure 2010 ('the Measure')). They also contain provision about the identification of relevant mental health service providers, and transitional provisions for patients who are already in secondary mental health services at the coming into force date of these Regulations.

2. Regulation 3 provides for the identification of a relevant mental health service provider in circumstances where a patient is using secondary mental health services provided by both a Local Health Board and a local authority.

3. Regulation 4 makes provision about the eligibility requirements which must be met before a person may be appointed as a care coordinator. Professional requirements which a person must satisfy are set out in Schedule 1.

4. Regulation 5 makes provision about the form and content of care and treatment plans. The form of a care and treatment plan is set out in Schedule 2, and is to be completed in the Welsh or the English language, or partly in Welsh and partly in English.

5. Regulation 6 makes provision about the persons who must be consulted by the care coordinator as part of the care coordinator's functions of preparing, reviewing and revising care and treatment plans. Provision is made also regarding persons who may be consulted by the care coordinator, and for the views of the patient to be taken into account before any consultation under this regulation takes place.

6. Regulation 7 provides for the review and revision of care and treatment plans. This includes provision about how frequently a plan must be reviewed and if necessary, revised, and who may request a review and, if necessary, revision.

7. Regulation 8 makes provision about the persons who must be provided with a

copy of a patient's care and treatment plan following the preparation, review or revision of that plan. Provision is made also regarding persons who may be provided with copies of such plans, for copies of plans to be withheld or only parts of copies to be provided, and for the views of the patient to be taken into account before any copies of plans or parts of plans are provided.

8. Regulation 9 makes provision about how copies of care and treatment plans are to be provided, and allows for the use of both electronic and non-electronic means of provision.

9. Regulation 10 makes provision about the information which is to be provided to an individual when he or she is discharged from secondary mental health services.

10. Regulation 11 makes transitional provision for patients who are already in secondary mental health services at the coming into force date of these Regulations. This includes provision for patients who do not have a care coordinator or a care and treatment plan at the coming into force date.

11. A regulatory impact assessment has been prepared as to the likely costs and benefits of complying with these Regulations. A copy can be obtained from the Mental Health Legislation Team, Department for Health, Social Services and Children, Welsh Government, Cathays Park, Cardiff CF10 3NQ.

A1.14 Forms for Use in Wales

The following forms can be downloaded from www.wales.nhs.uk/sites3/page.cfm?orgId=816&pid=33958.

Hospital Forms

- Form HO 1 Mental Health Act 1983, section 2 – application by Nearest Relative for admission for assessment;
- Form HO 2 Mental Health Act 1983, section 2 – application by an Approved Mental health Professional for admission for assessment;
- Form HO 3 Mental Health Act 1983, section 2 – joint medical recommendation for admission for assessment;
- Form HO 4 Mental Health Act 1983, section 2 – medical recommendation for admission for assessment;
- Form HO 5 Mental Health Act 1983, section 3 – application by nearest relative for admission for treatment;
- Form HO 6 Mental Health Act 1983, section 3 – application by an Approved Mental Health Professional for admission for treatment;
- Form HO 7 Mental Health Act 1983, section 3 – joint medical recommendation for admission for treatment;
- Form HO 8 Mental Health Act 1983, section 3 – medical recommendation for admission for treatment;
- Form HO 9 Mental Health Act 1983, section 4 – emergency application by NR for admission for assessment;
- Form HO 10 Mental Health Act 1983, section 4 – emergency application by an Approved Mental Health Professional for admission for assessment;
- Form HO 11 Mental Health Act 1983, section 4 – medical recommendation for emergency admission for assessment;
- Form HO 12 Mental Health Act 1983, section 5(2) – report on hospital in-patient;
- Form HO 13 Mental Health Act 1983 section 5(4) – record of hospital in-patient;
- Form HO 14 Mental Health Act 1983, sections 2, 3 and 4 – record of detention in hospital;
- Form HO 15 Mental Health Act 1983, section 20 – renewal of authority for detention;
- Form HO 16 Mental Health Act 1983, section 21B – authority for detention after absence without leave for more than 28 days;
- Form HO 17 Mental Health Act 1983, section 23 – discharge by the Responsible Clinician or the Hospital Managers.

Guardianship Forms
- Form GU 1 Mental Health Act 1983, section 7 – guardianship application by nearest relative;
- Form GU 2 Mental Health Act 1983, section 7 – guardianship application by an Approved Mental Health Professional;
- Form GU 3 Mental Health Act 1983, section 7 – joint medical recommendation for reception into guardianship;
- Form GU 4 Mental Health Act 1983, section 7 – medical recommendation for reception into guardianship;
- Form GU 5 Mental Health Act 1983, section 7 – record of acceptance of guardianship application;
- Form GU 6 Mental Health Act 1983, section 20 – renewal of authority for guardianship;
- Form GU 7 Mental Health Act 1983, section 21B – authority for guardianship after absence without leave for more than 28 days;
- Form GU 8 Mental Health Act 1983, section 23 – discharge by the Responsible Clinician or the responsible local social services authority.

Community Treatment Order Forms
- Form CP 1 Mental Health Act 1983, section 17A – CTO;
- Form CP 2 Mental Health Act 1983, section 17B – variation of conditions of a CTO
- Form CP 3 Mental Health Act 1983, section 20A – report extending the community treatment period
- Form CP 4 Mental Health Act 1983, section 21B – authority for community treatment after absence without leave for more than 28 days;
- Form CP 5 Mental Health Act 1983, section 17E – notice of recall to hospital;

- Form CP 6 Mental Health Act 1983, section 17E – record of patient's detention in hospital following recall;
- Form CP 7 Mental Health Act 1983, section 17F – revocation of a CTO;
- Form CP 8 Mental Health Act 1983, section 23 – discharge by the Responsible Clinician or the Hospital Managers.

Transfers
- Form TC 1 Mental Health Act 1983, section 19 – authority for transfer from one hospital to another under different managers;
- Form TC 2 Mental Health Act 1983, section 19 – authority for transfer from hospital to guardianship;
- Form TC 3 Mental Health Act 1983, section 19 – authority for transfer of a patient from the guardianship of one guardian to another;
- Form TC 4 Mental Health Act 1983, section 19 – authority for transfer from guardianship to hospital;
- Form TC 5 Mental Health Act 1983, section 19A – authority for assignment of responsibility for a community patient from one hospital to another under different managers;
- Form TC 6 Mental Health Act 1983, section 17F(2) – authority for transfer of recalled community patient to a hospital under different managers;
- Form TC 7 Mental Health Act 1983, Part 6 – date of reception of a patient to hospital or into guardianship in Wales;
- Form TC 8 Mental Health Act 1983, Part 6 – transfer of patient subject to compulsion in the community;
- Form Nearest Relative 1 Mental Health Act 1983, section 25 – report barring discharge by nearest relative.

Treatment Forms

- Form CO 1 Mental Health Act 1983, section 57 – certificate of consent to treatment and second opinion;
- Form CO 2 Mental Health Act 1983, section 58(3)(a) – certificate of consent to treatment;
- Form CO 3 Mental Health Act 1983, section 58(3)(b) – certificate of second opinion;
- Form CO 4 Mental Health Act 1983, section 58A(3)(c) – certificate of consent to treatment (patients at least 18 years of age);
- Form CO 5 Mental Health Act 1983, section 58A(4)(c) – certificate of consent to treatment and second opinion (patients under 18 years of age);
- Form CO 6 Mental Health Act 1983, section 58A(5) – certificate of second opinion (patients who are not capable of understanding the nature, purpose and likely effects of the treatment);
- Form CO 7 Mental Health Act 1983, Part 4A – certificate of appropriateness of treatment to be given to a community patient (Part 4A Certificate).

Appendix 2: Guidelines and Forms for England

A2.1 Conflicts of Interest

From Chapter 39 of the 2015 revision of the *Code of Practice: Mental Health Act 1983*:[1]

Financial conflict

4. The current regulations require that where the patient is to be admitted to an independent hospital and the doctor providing one of the medical recommendations is on the staff of that hospital, the other medical recommendation must be given by a doctor who is not on the staff of that hospital. That is, there will be a potential conflict if both doctors giving recommendations are on the staff of the independent hospital. It is also good practice for doctors on the staff of an NHS trust or NHS foundation trust to ensure that one of the recommendations is given by a doctor not on the staff of that trust.

5. It may be beneficial for providers (NHS trusts, foundation trusts and the independent sector) in close proximity to organise a list of doctors who are available to provide a second recommendation.

6. An assessor will have a conflict of interest for financial reasons if the assessor stands to make a financial benefit (or loss) from their decision. There will not be a potential conflict of interest for financial reasons where an assessor is paid a fee for making an application or giving a medical recommendation if it is paid regardless of the outcome of the assessment.

7. An assessor will have a potential conflict of interest if both that assessor and one of the other assessors, the patient or the nearest relative (if the nearest relative is the applicant) are closely involved in the same business venture. Being closely involved is not defined in the regulations, but examples could include being a partner in a partnership, being a director or other office-holder of a company, or being a major shareholder in it. This will apply even if the business venture is not associated with the provision of services for the care and treatment of persons with a mental disorder.

8. Business ventures include any form of commercial enterprise from which the person concerned stands to profit. Such people include: directors and major investors in a company (of any size) which provides goods or services for profit; partners in a GP practice; partners in a business established as a limited liability partnership. Involvement in a business venture does not include involvement in societies and similar organisations which are essentially non-commercial, and from which the people concerned do not stand to profit.

Professional conflict

9. Regulations set out that a conflict of interest for professional reasons will occur where:

   • the assessor is in a line management or employment relationship with one of the other assessors or the patient or the nearest relative (where the nearest relative is the applicant);

- the assessor is a member of the same team as the patient; or
- where there are three assessors, all of them are members of the same team.

10. A line management relationship will exist whether an assessor manages, or is managed by, one of the other assessors, the patient or the nearest relative (where the nearest relative is the applicant). Similarly an employment relationship will exist whether the assessor employs, or is employed by, one of the other assessors, the patient or the nearest relative (where the nearest relative is the applicant).

11. For the purposes of the regulations a team is defined as a group of professionals who work together for clinical purposes on a routine basis. That might include a community mental health team, a crisis resolution or home treatment team, or staff on an in-patient unit (but not necessarily the staff of an entire hospital).

Urgent necessity

12. If there is a case of urgent necessity all three assessors may be from the same team. However, this should happen only in a genuine emergency, where the patient's need for urgent assessment outweighs the desirability of waiting for another assessor who has no potential conflict of interest. Any decisions made to proceed despite a potential conflict of interest should be recorded, with reasons, in case notes.

13. In a case of urgent necessity it is preferable to proceed with three assessors, despite a potential conflict of interest, rather than make the application under section 4 of the Act with only two assessors (one doctor and one Approved Mental Health Professional) (see paragraphs 15.6–15.8).

14. There are no other circumstances in which potential conflict of interest can be set aside because of urgent necessity.

A2.2 Forms for England

The following forms can be downloaded from www.mentalhealthlaw.co.uk/Mental_Health_Act_1983_Statutory_Forms.

Admission Forms

- Form A1 Mental Health Act 1983, section 2 – application by nearest relative for admission for assessment;
- Form A2 Mental Health Act 1983, section 2 – application by an Approved Mental Health Professional for admission for assessment;
- Form A3 Mental Health Act 1983, section 2 – joint medical recommendation for admission for assessment;
- Form A4 Mental Health Act 1983, section 2 – medical recommendation for admission for assessment;
- Form A5 Mental Health Act 1983, section 3 – application by nearest relative for admission for treatment;
- Form A6 Mental Health Act 1983, section 3 – application by an Approved Mental Health Professional for admission for treatment;
- Form A7 Mental Health Act 1983, section 3 – joint medical recommendation for admission for treatment;
- Form A8 Mental Health Act 1983, section 3 – medical recommendation for admission for treatment;
- Form A9 Mental Health Act 1983, section 4 – emergency application by nearest relative for admission for assessment;
- Form A10 Mental Health Act 1983, section 4 – emergency application by an Approved Mental Health Professional for admission for assessment;
- Form A11 Mental Health Act 1983, section 4 – medical recommendation for emergency admission for assessment.

Hospital Forms

- Form H1 Mental Health Act 1983, section 5(2) – report on hospital in-patient;
- Form H2 Mental Health Act 1983, section 5(4) – record of hospital in-patient;
- Form H3 Mental Health Act 1983, sections 2, 3 and 4 – record of detention in hospital;
- Form H4 Mental Health Act 1983, section 19 – authority for transfer from one hospital to another under different managers;
- Form H5 Mental Health Act 1983, section 20 – renewal of authority for detention;
- Form H6 Mental Health Act 1983, section 21B – authority for detention after absence without leave for more than 28 days.

Guardianship Forms

- Form G1 Mental Health Act 1983, section 7 – guardianship application by nearest relative;
- Form G2 Mental Health Act 1983, section 7 – guardianship application by an Approved Mental Health Professional;
- Form G3 Mental Health Act 1983, section 7 – joint medical recommendation for reception into guardianship;
- Form G4 Mental Health Act 1983, section 7 – medical recommendation for reception into guardianship;
- Form G5 Mental Health Act 1983, section 7 – record of acceptance of guardianship application;
- Form G6 Mental Health Act 1983, section 19 – authority for transfer from hospital to guardianship;
- Form G7 Mental Health Act 1983, section 19 – authority for transfer of a patient from the guardianship of one guardian to another;
- Form G8 Mental Health Act 1983, section 19 – authority for transfer from guardianship to hospital;
- Form G9 Mental Health Act 1983, section 20 – renewal of authority for guardianship;
- Form G10 Mental Health Act 1983, section 21B – authority for guardianship after absence without leave for more than 28 days.

Miscellaneous Forms

- Form M1 Part 6 – date of reception of a patient in England;
- Form M2 Mental Health Act 1983, section 25 – report barring discharge by nearest relative.

Treatment Forms

- Form T1 – Mental Health Act 1983, section 57 – certificate of consent to treatment and second opinion;
- Form T2 – Mental Health Act 1983, section 58 – certificate of consent to treatment;
- Form T3 – Mental Health Act 1983, section 58(3)(b) – certificate of second opinion;
- Form T4 – Mental Health Act 1983, section 58A(3) – certificate of consent to treatment (patients at least 18 years old);
- Form T5 – Mental Health Act 1983, section 58A(4) – certificate of consent to treatment and second opinion (patients under the age of 18);
- Form T6 – Mental Health Act 1983, section 58A(5) – certificate of second opinion (patients who are not capable of understanding the nature, purpose and likely effects of the treatment).

Community Treatment Order Forms

- Form CTO1 Mental Health Act 1983, section 17A – CTO;
- Form CTO2 Mental Health Act 1983, section 17B – variation of conditions of a CTO;
- Form CTO3 Mental Health Act 1983, section 17E – CTO – notice of recall to hospital;
- Form CTO4 Mental Health Act 1983, section 17E – CTO – record of patient's detention in hospital after recall;
- Form CTO5 Mental Health Act 1983, section 17F(4) – revocation of CTO;
- Form CTO6 Mental Health Act 1983, section 17F(2) – authority for transfer of recalled community patient to a hospital under different managers;
- Form CTO7 Mental Health Act 1983, section 20A – CTO – report extending the community treatment period;
- Form CTO8 Mental Health Act 1983, section 21B – authority for extension of community treatment period after absence without leave for more than 28 days;
- Form CTO9 Part 6 – community patients transferred to England;
- Form CTO10 Mental Health Act 1983, section 19A – authority for assignment of responsibility for community patient to hospital under different managers;
- Form CTO11 Mental Health Act 1983, section 64C(4) – certificate of appropriateness of treatment to be given to community patient (Part 4A certificate);
- Form CTO12 Regulation 28(1A) Mental Health Act 1983, section 64C(4A) – certificate that community patient has capacity to consent (or if under 16 is competent to consent) to treatment and has done so (Part 4A consent certificate).

References

Chapter 1

1 Department of Health, *Code of Practice: Mental Health Act 1983* (The Stationery Office, 2015).

2 Welsh Assembly Government, *Mental Health Act 1983: Code of Practice for Wales* (The Stationery Office, 2016).

3 Department for Constitutional Affairs, *Mental Capacity Act 2005: Code of Practice* (The Stationery Office, 2007).

4 Ministry of Justice, *Mental Capacity Act 2005: Deprivation of Liberty Safeguards. Code of Practice to Supplement the Main Mental Capacity Act 2005 Code of Practice* (The Stationery Office, 2008).

5 Department of Health, *Reference Guide to the Mental Health Act 1983* (The Stationery Office, 2015).

6 Secretary of State for Health, *Mental Health Act 1983: Instructions with Respect to the Exercise of Approval Functions 2014* (Department of Health, 2014).

7 *Statutory Instruments 2008 No. 2699 (L. 16): The Tribunal Procedure (First-Tier Tribunal) (Health, Education and Social Care Chamber) Rules 2008* (The Stationery Office).

8 *Re. F (Mental Health Sterilisation)* [1990] 2 AC 1 HL.

9 *Ibid.*

10 *R. (on the application of Lee-Hirons) v. Secretary of State for Justice (on the application of Wooder) v. Feggetter* [2002] All ER (D) 243.

11 *Black v. Forsey* [1988] SC (HL) 28.

12 *Devon County Council v. Hawkins* [1967] 2 QB 26; 1 All ER 235.

13 *B v. Croydon Health Authority* [1995] 1 All ER 683.

14 *R. v. Hallstrom* [1986] 2 All ER 306.

15 *Ibid.*

16 *B v. Barking, Havering and Brentwood Community Healthcare NHS Trust* (1999) 47 BMLR 112.

17 *R. (on the application of DR) v. Mersey Care NHS Trust* (2002) EWHC 1810.

18 *KL v. Somerset Partnership NHS Foundation Trust* [2011] UKUT 233 (AAC).

19 *SL v. Ludlow Street Healthcare* (2015) UKUT 398 (AAC).

20 Statement on Article 14 of the Convention on the Rights of Persons with Disabilities, September 2014, www.ohchr.org/EN/NewsEvents/Pages/DisplayNews.aspx?NewsID=15183.

21 Committee on the Rights of Persons with Disabilities: Concluding observations on the initial report of the United Kingdom of Great Britain and Northern Ireland, October 2017.

22 The United Kingdom Government Response to the Report by the United Nations Committee on the Rights of Persons with Disabilities under article 6 of the Optional Protocol to the Convention, June 2018.

23 A. S. Zigmond, 'Medical Incapacity Act', *Psychiatric Bulletin*, 22 (1998), 657–8.

Chapter 2

1 *Statutory Instruments 2001 No. 3712: The Mental Health Act 1983 (Remedial) Order 2001: Mental Health, England and Wales* (The Stationery Office).

2 *Fernandes de Oliveira v. Portugal* [2019] ECHR App. No. 78103/14.

3 *Savage v. South Essex Partnership NHS Foundation Trust* [2010] EWHC 865 (QB).

4 *Rabone and another (Appellants) v. Pennine Care NHS Foundation Trust (Respondent)* [2012] UKSC 2.

5 *Osman v. UK* (2000) 29 EHRR 245.

6   *Aftanache* v. *Romania* [2020] ECHR 339.

7   *Savage* (n. 3 above).

8   *Rabone* (n. 4 above).

9   G. Szmukler, G. Richardson and G. Owen, ' "Rabone" and Four Unresolved Problems in Mental Health Law', *Psychiatrist*, 37 (2013), 297–301.

10   *Fernandes de Oliveira* (n. 2 above).

11   *Re. A (Children) (conjoined twins)* [2000] 4 All ER 961.

12   *Jalloh* v. *Germany* 2006 EHRR 667.

13   *Herczegfalvy* v. *Austria (A/242-B)* (1993) 15 EHRR 437, ECHR.

14   *JK* v. *A Local Health Board* [2019] EWHC 67 (Fam).

15   *Keenan* v. *UK* (2001) 33 EHRR 913.

16   *MS* v. *UK 24527/08* [2012] ECHR 804.

17   *HL* v. *UK (45508/99)* (2005) 40 EHRR 32; (2004) MHLR 236, ECHR.

18   *Ibid.*

19   *Ibid.*

20   *Winterwerp* v. *The Netherlands* (1979) 2 EHRR 387.

21   *R. (on the application of MH)* v. *Secretary of State for Health* [2005] UKHL 60.

22   *MH* v. *UK – 11577/06 – Chamber Judgment* [2013] ECHR 1008.

23   *R (OK)* v. *FTT* [2017] UKUT 22 (AAC).

24   *London Borough of Hillingdon* v. *Neary and another* [2011] EWHC 1377 (COP).

25   *R. (G)* v. *Nottinghamshire Healthcare NHS Trust* [2008] EWHC 1096.

26   *R. (on the application of B)* v. *(1) Dr SS Responsible Medical Officer, Broadmoor Hospital (2) Dr G Second Opinion Appointed Doctor (3) Secretary of State for the Department of Health* [2005] EWHC 1936 (Admin).

27   *AG* v. *BMBC and another* [2016] EWCOP 37.

28   *An NHS Trust* v. *XB* [2020] EWCOP 71.

29   *Storck* v. *Germany – 61603/00* [2005] ECHR 406.

30   *Savage* (n. 3 above).

Chapter 3

1   *Re. B (Adult: Refusal of Medical Treatment)* [2002] 2 All ER 449.

2   *Sidaway* v. *Board of Governors of the Bethlem Royal Hospital* [1985] 1 All ER 643.

3   *Heart of England NHS Foundation Trust* v. *JB* [2014] EWHC 342 (COP).

4   *Chatterton* v. *Gerson* [1981] 1 All ER 257.

5   General Medical Council, *Guidance of Professional Standards and Ethics for Doctors: Decision Making and Consent* (2020).

6   *Bolam* v. *Friern Hospital Management Committee* [1957] 1 WLR 583, 587.

7   *Bolitho* v. *City and Hackney HA* [1997] 4 All ER 771.

8   *Montgomery* v. *Lanarkshire Health Board* [2015] UKSC 11.

9   *Re. R (A Minor) (Wardship: Medical Treatment)* [1992] Fam 11; [1991] 4 All ER 177, CA.

10   Practice Direction First-Tier Tribunal Health and Social Care Chamber Statements and Reports in Mental Health Cases 2013.

11   K. A. Ruck and C. Auckland, 'More Presumptions Please? Wishes, Feelings and Best Interest Decision-Making', *Elder Law Journal* (2015), 293–301.

12   *X Primary Care Trust* v. *XB and another* [2012] EWHC 1390 (Fam).

13   *Cheshire West and Chester Council* v. *P* (2014) UKSC 19.

14   *Ibid.*

15   *ZH (by his Litigation Friend)* v. *Metropolitan Police Commissioner* [2012] All ER (D) 134.

16   *HL* v. *United Kingdom (45508/99)* (2005) 40 EHRR 32; (2004) MHLR 236, ECHR.

17   House of Lords Select Committee on the Mental Capacity Act 2005, *Mental Capacity Act 2005: Post-Legislative Scrutiny (HL 139, Report of Session 2013–14)* (The Stationery Office, 2014).

18 N. Brindle and T. Branton, 'Interface between the Mental Health Act and Mental Capacity Act: The Deprivation of Liberty Safeguards', *Advances in Psychiatric Treatment*, 16 (2010), 430–7.

19 *AM v. (1) South London & Maudsley NHS Foundation Trust and (2) The Secretary of State for Health* [2013] UKUT 0365 (AAC).

20 *Cheshire West* (n. 13 above).

21 Reforming the Mental Health Act. Government response to consultation, July 2021.

22 *GJ v. The Foundation Trust and others* [2009] EWHC 2972 (Fam).

23 *AM* (n. 19 above).

24 *A PCT v. LDV* [2013] EWHC 272 (Fam).

25 Ministry of Justice, *Mental Capacity Act 2005: Deprivation of Liberty Safeguards. Code of Practice to Supplement the Main Mental Capacity Act 2005 Code of Practice* (The Stationery Office, 2008).

26 *DCC v. KH* (2009) COP 11729380.

27 *R. (Ferreira) HM Senior Coroner for Inner South London and others* [2017] EWCA Civ 3.

28 *Christine Esegbona (deceased) v. King's College Hospital NHS Foundation Trust* [2019] EWHC 77 (QB).

29 *An NHS Trust v. Dr A* (2013) EWHC 2442 (COP).

30 *Re. R (A Minor)* (n. 9 above).

31 *A Local Health Board v. AB (Rev. 1)* [2015] EWCOP 31.

32 DoLS Code of Practice.

Chapter 4

1 Department of Health, *Code of Practice: Mental Health Act 1983* (The Stationery Office, 2015).

2 Welsh Assembly Government, *Mental Health Act 1983: Code of Practice for Wales* (The Stationery Office, 2016).

Chapter 5

1 Department of Health, *Code of Practice: Mental Health Act 1983* (The Stationery Office, 2015); Welsh Assembly

Government, *Mental Health Act 1983: Code of Practice for Wales* (The Stationery Office, 2016).

2 *R. v. Mental Health Review Tribunal for the South Thames Region, ex p. Smith* [1998] EWHC 832.

3 *DN v. Northumberland Tyne and Wear NHS Foundation Trust* (2011) UKUT 327 (AAC).

4 *H-L v. Partnerships in Care and Secretary of State for Justice* [2013] UKUT 500 (AAC).

5 *WH v. Llanarth Court Hospital (Partnerships in Care)* [2015] UKUT 0695 (AAC).

6 *MD v. Mersey Care NHS Trust* [2013] UKUT 0127(AAC).

7 *Ibid.*

8 *Devon Partnership NHS Trust v. SSHSC* [2021] EWHC 101 (Admin).

9 *Townley v. Rushworth* (1963) 62 LGR 95.

10 Statutory Instruments 2008 No. 1205: The Mental Health (Conflicts of Interest) (England) Regulations 2008 (The Stationery Office).

11 Statutory Instruments 2008 No. 2440: The Mental Health (Conflicts of Interest) (Wales) Regulations 2008 (The Stationery Office).

12 Department of Health, *Reference Guide to the Mental Health Act 1983* (The Stationery Office, 2015).

13 *R. (on the application of DR) v. Mersey Care NHS Trust* (2002) EWHC 1810.

14 *R. (Sessay) v. South London and Maudsley NHS Foundation Trust and The Commissioner for Police for the Metropolis* [2011] EWHC 2617 (QB).

15 Home Office, *Guidance for the Implementation of Changes to Police Powers and Places of Safety Provisions in the Mental Health Act 1983* (2017).

16 The Mental Health (Hospital, Guardianship and Treatment) (England) (Amendment) Regulations 2020.

17 See www.gov.uk/government/ publications/electronic-communication-

of-statutory-forms-under-the-mental-health-act.

18 *Rabone and another (Appellants)*
    v. *Pennine Care NHS Foundation Trust*
    (Respondent) [2012] UKSC 2.

19 Great Britain Parliament Joint
    Committee on Human Rights, *Legislative*
    Scrutiny: Mental Health Bill. Fourth
    Report of Session 2006–07 (The Stationery
    Office, 2007).

20 Great Britain Parliament Joint
    Committee on Human Rights, *Legislative*
    Scrutiny: Seventh Progress Report.
    Fifteenth Report of Session 2006–07 (The
    Stationery Office, 2007).

21 *NL* v. *Hampshire CC* [2014] UKUT 475
    (AAC).

22 See www.legislation.gov.uk/ukpga/2018/
    27/enacted.

23 Mental Health Units (Use of Force) Act
    2018: Statutory Guidance for NHS
    Organisations, May 2021.

Chapter 6

1   In the Central Criminal Court. Mrs
    Justice McGowan. *Regina* v. *Jonty*
    Bravery. Sentence.

2   *SSJ* v. *RB* [2011] EWCA Civ 1608.

3   *Secretary of State for Justice* v. *MM* [2018]
    UKSC 60.

4   HM Prison and Probation Service (2019)
    Guidance: Discharge Conditions that
    Amount to Deprivation of Liberty.

5   *Hertfordshire County Council* v. *AB*
    [2018] EWHC 3103 (Fam).

6   *County Council* v. *ZZ* [2013] COPLR 463.

7   *Birmingham CC* v. *SR; Lancashire CC*
    v. *JTA* [2019] EWCOP 28.

8   *DB* v. *Betsi Cadwaldr University Health*
    Board [2021] UKUT 53.

Chapter 7

1   Lord Warner, Hansard HL, vol. 688, part
    28, cols 702 and 703 (17 January 2007).

2   Department of Health, *Code of Practice:*
    Mental Health Act 1983 (The Stationery
    Office, 2015).

3   *MP* v. *Mersey Care NHS Trust* (2011)
    UKUT 107 (AAC).

4   *Welsh Ministers* v. *PJ* [2018] UKSC 66.

5   Care Quality Commission, *Monitoring*
    the Use of the Mental Health Act in 2009/
    10: The Care Quality Commission's First
    Report on the Exercise of Its Functions in
    Keeping under Review the Operation of the
    Mental Health Act 1983 (CQC, 2010),
    p. 62.

6   *LW* v. *Cornwall Partnership NHS*
    Foundation Trust [2018] UKUT 408
    (AAC).

7   *CM* v. *Derbyshire Healthcare NHS*
    Foundation Trust [2011] UKUT 129
    (AAC) (emphasis added).

Chapter 8

1   *Re. AA* (2012) EWHC 4378 (COP);
    (2012) MHLO 182.

2   *B* v. *Croydon Health Authority* [1995]
    1 All ER 683.

3   *Nottinghamshire Healthcare NHS Trust*
    v. *RC* (2014) EWCOP 1317.

4   *A Midlands NHS Trust* v. *RD* [2021]
    EWCOP 35.

5   *Ibid.*

6   *A Mental Health Trust* v. *ER* [2021]
    EWCOP 32.

7   *Re. H (Mental patients:*
    diagnosis) (1992) FLR Jul 1; [1993]
    1, 28–33.

8   *A Healthcare and B NHS Trust* v. *CC*
    (2020) EWHC 574 (Fam).

9   *Re. C (Adult refusal of medical treatment)*
    [1994] 1 All ER 819.

10 *Re. MB (Adult, medical treatment)* [1997]
    38 BMLR 175 CA.

11 *Tameside & Glossop Acute Services Unit*
    v. *CH (a patient)* [1996] 1 FLR 762.

12 *Re. C* (n. 9 above).

13 *St George's Healthcare NHS Trust* v. *S;*
    R. v. *Collins and others, ex p. S* [1998]
    3 All ER 673.

14 *NHS Trust and others* v. *FG* [2014]
    EWCOP 30.

15 *Guys & St Thomas' NHS Foundation Trust & South London and Maudsley NHS Foundation Trust* v. *R.* [2020] EWCOP 4.

16 Department of Health, *Code of Practice: Mental Health Act 1983* (The Stationery Office, 2015).

17 *RM* v. *St Andrew's Healthcare* [2010] UKUT 119 (AAC), HM/0837/2010.

18 M. Kinton, K. Dudleston, P. Jefferys, *et al.* 'Medication for Side-Effects under the Mental Health Act', *Psychiatrist*, 32 (2008), 358.

19 Care Quality Commission, *Monitoring the Use of the Mental Health Act in 2009/ 10: The Care Quality Commission's First Report on the Exercise of Its Functions in Keeping under Review the Operation of the Mental Health Act 1983* (CQC, 2010).

Chapter 9

1 *R.* v. *Riverside Mental Health Trust, ex p. Huzzey* [1998] 43 BMLR 167.

2 *Statutory Instruments 2008 No. 2699 (L. 16): The Tribunal Procedure (First-tier Tribunal) (Health, Education and Social Care Chamber) Rules 2008* (The Stationery Office); *Statutory Instruments 2008 No. 2705 (L. 17): The Mental Health Review Tribunal for Wales Rules 2008* (The Stationery Office); R. Carnwath, *Practice Direction: First-Tier and Upper Tribunal. Use of The Welsh Language in Tribunals in Wales* (Tribunals Judiciary, 2008), www.judiciary.uk/wp-content/uploads/JCO/Documents/Practice+Directions/Tribunals/UseoftheWelshlanguage.pdf.

3 *GM* v. *Dorset Healthcare National Health Service Trust and the Secretary of State for Justice* [2020] UKUT 152 (AAC).

4 *VS* v. *St Andrews Healthcare* [2018] UKUT 250.

5 *SM* v. *Livewell Southwest CIC* [2020] UKUT 191 (AAC).

6 *YA* v. *Central and North West London NHS Trust and others* [2015] UKUT 37 (AAC).

7 *R. (OK)* v. *FTT* [2017] UKUT 22 (AAC).

8 *PI* v. *West London Mental Health NHS Trust* [2017] UKUT 66 (AAC).

9 J. Sullivan, *Practice Direction: First-Tier Tribunal, Health Education and Social Care Chamber, Statements and Reports in Mental Health Cases* (Tribunals Judiciary, 2013).

10 Mental Health Law Online, *Tribunal Procedure: Failure to Submit Reports to the Tribunal on Time (17 April 2015) (2015) MHLO 38* (2015), www.mentalhealthlaw.co.uk.

11 Sullivan, Practice Direction (n. 9 above).

12 *Statutory Instruments 2008 No. 2699 (L. 16): The Tribunal Procedure (First-tier Tribunal) (Health, Education and Social Care Chamber) Rules 2008* (The Stationery Office).

13 *GB* v. *South West London & St George's MH NHS Trust* [2013] UKUT 58 (AAC).

14 *AH* v. *West London MH NHS Trust* (2010) UKUT 264 (AAC).

15 *AH* v. *West London MH NHS Trust and SoS (J) (Final)* (2011) UKUT 74 (AAC).

16 Department for Constitutional Affairs, *Mental Capacity Act 2005: Code of Practice* (The Stationery Office, 2007).

17 *R. (B)* v. *MHRT* (2002) All ER (D) 304 (Jul).

18 *Winterwerp* v. *The Netherlands* (1979) 2 EHRR 387.

19 Department of Health, *Code of Practice: Mental Health Act 1983* (The Stationery Office, 2015).

20 *CM* v. *Derbyshire Healthcare NHS Foundation Trust* [2011] UKUT 129 (AAC).

21 *R.* v. *East London and the City Mental Health Trust, ex p. von Brandenburg* [2003] UKHL 58; [2004] 1 All ER 400.

22 *R. (Zhang)* v. *Whittington Hospital* (2013) EWHC 358 (Admin); (2013) MHLO 29.

Chapter 10

1 Department of Health, *Code of Practice: Mental Health Act 1983* (The Stationery Office, 2015).

2 *Re. W (a minor) (medical treatment)* [1992] 4 All ER 627.

3 *An NHS Foundation Hospital* v. *P* (2014) EWHC 1650 (Fam).

4   *Gillick* v. *Norfolk and Wisbech Area Health Authority* [1985] 3 All ER 402.

5   *Ibid.*

6   *R. (on the application of Axon)* v. *Secretary of State for Health* [2006] EWHC 37 (Admin).

7   *NHS Trust* v. *X (No. 2)* [2021] EWHC 65.

8   *Re. D (A Child; Deprivation of Liberty)* [2015] EWHC 922 (Fam).

9   *D (A Child)* [2019] UKSC 42.

Chapter 11

1   Secretary of State for Health, *Mental Health Act 1983: Instructions with Respect to the Exercise of Approval Functions 2014* (Department of Health, 2014).

2   *Ibid.*

3   J. Munby, *What Price Dignity? Keynote Address by Lord Justice Munby to The LAG Community Care Conference: Protecting Liberties on 14 July 2010* (Legal Action Group, 2010).

Chapter 12

1   Modernising the Mental Health Act. Increasing Choice, Reducing Compulsion. Final report of the Independent Review of the Mental Health Act 1983, December 2018.

2   Reforming the Mental Health Act. Presented to Parliament by the Secretary of State for Health and Social Care and the Lord Chancellor and Secretary of State for Justice by Command of Her Majesty, January 2021.

3   Reforming the Mental Health Act. Government Response to Consultation. Presented to Parliament by the Secretary of State for Health and Social Care and the Lord Chancellor and Secretary of State for Justice by Command of Her Majesty, July 2021.

4   Legal Guidance for Mental Health, Learning Disability and Autism, and Specialised Commissioning Services Supporting People of All Ages During the Coronavirus Pandemic, May 2020.

5   COVID-19: Interim Methodology for Second Opinions. Care Quality Commission, March 2020.

6   Mental Health Tribunal Response to Covid-19 Emergency. Update April 2021.

Appendix 1

1   National Assembly for Wales, *Proposed Mental Health (Wales) Measure 2010 [As Passed]* (2010), https://gov.wales/sites/default/files/publications/2019-03/mental-health-act-1983-approval-of-approved-clinicians-wales-july-2018.pdf.

2   *Statutory Instruments 2008 No. 2705 (L. 17): The Mental Health Review Tribunal for Wales Rules 2008* (The Stationery Office).

3   R. Carnwath, *Practice Direction: First-Tier and Upper Tribunal. Use of The Welsh Language in Tribunals in Wales* (Tribunals Judiciary, 2008), www.judiciary.uk/wp-content/uploads/JCO/Documents/Practice+Directions/Tribunals/UseoftheWelshlanguage.pdf.

4   Bwrdd lechyd Prifysgol Betsi Cadwaldr University Health Board, *Mental Health Act 1983 Section 12(2): Approval / Re Approval Process and Criteria for Wales* (January 2022).

5   Welsh Ministers, *National Health Service (Wales) Act 2006: Mental Health Act 1983 Approved Clinician (Wales) Directions 2008* (The Stationery Office, 2008), www.mentalhealthlaw.co.uk/Mental_Health_Act_1983_Approved_Clinician_(Wales)_Directions_2008.

6   Welsh Assembly Government, *Mental Health Act 1983: Approval of Approved Clinicians in Wales* (Welsh Government, 2011), https://gov.wales/sites/default/files/publications/2019-03/mental-health-act-1983-approval-of-approved-clinicians-wales-july-2018.pdf.

7   *Statutory Instruments 2011 No. 2942 (W.318): Mental Health (Care Co-ordination and Care and Treatment Planning) (Wales) Regulations 2011* (The Stationery Office).

Index

Printed in the United States
by Baker & Taylor Publisher Services